Quantum
DNA
HEALING

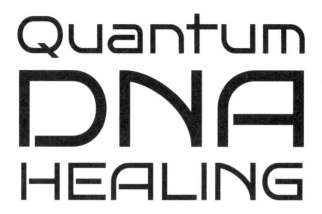

Quantum DNA HEALING

Consciousness Techniques for
Altering Your Genetic Destiny

ALTHEA S. HAWK

Bear & Company
Rochester, Vermont • Toronto, Canada

Bear & Company
One Park Street
Rochester, Vermont 05767
www.BearandCompanyBooks.com

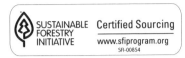

Text stock is SFI certified

Bear & Company is a division of Inner Traditions International

Library of Congress Cataloging-in-Publication Data
Names: Hawk, Althea S., author.
Title: Quantum DNA healing : consciousness techniques for altering your genetic destiny / Althea S. Hawk.
Description: Rochester, Vermont : Bear & Company, [2017] | Includes bibliographical references and index.
Identifiers: LCCN 2016037739 (print) | LCCN 2016048702 (e-book) | ISBN 9781591432876 (paperback) | ISBN 9781591432906 (e-book)
Subjects: LCSH: Genetic regulation. | Holistic medicine. | Mind and body. | BISAC: BODY, MIND & SPIRIT / Healing / Energy (Chi Kung, Reiki, Polarity). | HEALTH & FITNESS / Alternative Therapies. | MEDICAL / Alternative Medicine.
Classification: LCC QH450 .H38 2017 (print) | LCC QH450 (e-book) | DDC 572.8/65—dc23
LC record available at https://lccn.loc.gov/2016037739

Printed and bound in the United States by Lake Book Manufacturing, Inc. The text stock is SFI certified. The Sustainable Forestry Initiative® program promotes sustainable forest management.

10 9 8 7 6 5 4 3 2 1

Text design by Debbie Glogover and layout by Priscilla Baker
This book was typeset in Garamond Premier Pro with Bruno Ace and Gill Sans used as display typefaces

Cover images courtesy of Shutterstock

To send correspondence to the author of this book, mail a first-class letter to the author c/o Inner Traditions • Bear & Company, One Park Street, Rochester, VT 05767, and we will forward the communication, or contact the author directly through her website, **altheahawk.com**.

This book has many co-creators, from both the physical and nonphysical realms, who assisted me in bringing it forward, along with the gift to humanity its message conveys. I am truly humbled by the guidance, wisdom, and the unconditional love we are offered on our journeys to heal and grow, to fulfill our divine purpose and carry out our life's work. Each has contributed something unique and invaluable to the birth of new energies and expanded consciousness, individually and to the collective; to my personal evolution and healing; as well as to the manifestation of new understanding and this body of work. My heartfelt gratitude is extended to all of them, and to Grant in particular, for helping me with all that was needed in order for me to tell this story.

Contents

⊃⊂

Erasing the Imprint
of Disease

*We have to remember that what we observe is not nature
in itself, but nature exposed to our method of questioning.*

WERNER HEISENBERG,
PHYSICS AND PHILOSOPHY[1]

What follows is a chronicle of the healing journey that led me back, not
only to a significantly improved state of health and vitality, but more fundamentally, from the brink of a precarious state of existence associated
with life-threatening physiological impairment and disease. My return
occurred after many years of physical compromise and infirmity, punctu-
ated by brief periods of reprieve, only to be followed by those that were
even more unremitting and potentially grave. However, this is not a book
about my suffering, as real and perhaps dire as my challenges were at
times, but one that describes an outcome to the journey by rather unex-
pected and unlikely means. It is a story about change and the opportunity
that my circumstances present to others, patients and practitioners alike.
It is one that I believe has tremendous potential in the spheres of medical
science and healing modalities and that I feel compelled to share.

It is a journey about how I changed my biology and genetic coding by altering my DNA in a unique way and, in doing so, erased the

imprint of illness and disease that had been my reality for the better part of the last decade or so. This is the kind of claim that could easily generate controversy among many—practitioners, scientists, patients, and even ethicists. It becomes particularly interesting when the circumstances that surround my case cannot wholly be explained by the current understanding of genetics, mechanisms of disease, nor the principles of modern science in the physical sense. These challenges were compounded by the fact that many of the changes that occurred at more subtle, nonphysical levels, as a result of specific therapeutic techniques employed to this end, cannot be measured by medical or scientific means at this time. As has been so aptly stated, "for the modern mind, a credible explanation is a scientific explanation."[2]

Over the years, my health situation unraveled and worsened. This was largely due to the fact that many of my conditions including a cellular disorder, cancer, a number of skeletal tumors, heavy metal toxicity, and an inflammatory condition had remained undiagnosed for extremely long periods of time, well after many of the symptoms were very apparent. Unfortunately, these had all evaded my conventional-medicine medical practitioners, until it was almost too late. By this point, I was physically compromised and energetically depleted. Most of the therapies and treatments I had tried were unsuccessful in relieving my symptoms, much less in promoting healing. My sense was telling me that the answer to my survival and improvement in health resided in something different than anything I had tried so far or was currently available. As I read, researched, and came to understand the mechanisms of my own disease and genetics in a different light, it became apparent to me that the therapeutic and pharmacological approaches I was undertaking at the time held little promise for healing. The journey that ensued in the aftermath of this realization has allowed me to investigate and make sense of the critical connection between aspects of the physical and the nonphysical world, in order to create a more complete picture of who we are at the genetic level, how we become ill, and how we can heal.

The basis for the guidance I received and much of the material contained in this book came from repositories or dimensions of consciousness in the etheric, nonordinary realms, through a series of personal spiritual journeys and channels. These included the Akashic Records and other less publicly known archives of spiritual and esoteric knowledge. Information of this nature is received outside the capacity of normal human consciousness and requires some translation through the brain's limbic system into language and perception that is recognizable and understood by us. With some training, it is possible to set aside preconceived notions and bias and, without the involvement of the conscious mind, receive information on almost any subject (depending on our level of consciousness), as long as it is requested for our best and highest good, or for the good of others, as I have done here. Depending on the particular repository of knowledge within which I am working, some journeys or channeled information may be received as regular English language that is reasonably clear; other times it is a little more cryptic or is fed to me in smaller sound bites of information as words or small phrases. Messages conveyed without words in the form of sensory metaphors appear as visual images or sounds that embody the intent of the message and tell the story. As Ervin Laszlo, leading systems theorist and Nobel Peace Prize nominee, points out:

Today the Western world takes as real only that which is actually to hand—which is "manifest." People dismiss ideas of a wider sphere of reality and consider experiences of it as a mere fantasy. Because what modern people see is constrained by what they believe they can see, everything that's not conveyed to the mind by the eye and ear is missing from the modern view of the world. Experiences of a deeper or higher sphere of reality are confined to the subconscious regions of the mind and recognized only in esthetic, mystical, or religious exaltation; in love; and in sexual union. In the everyday context the intuitions conveyed by such experiences are ascribed to the unfathomable intuition of artists, poets, prophets, and gurus.[3]

The information contained in this book and the profound results that were achieved in my efforts to heal demonstrate that we are truly inseparable from these nonordinary realms. As some are only recently beginning to appreciate, reality cannot be adequately explained within a three-dimensional context. It irrevocably exists beyond our senses and our physicality, yet we have an ability to contact and communicate in these realms in a very real way for guidance, information, and healing.

This source of knowledge ultimately led me to what I believe is the truth about our genetics and down the path of healing by re-encoding my genes. By *re-encoding*, I mean more than simply modifying genetic expression, which is the process by which DNA instructions are utilized to synthesize gene products for the purposes of biological regulation and function in the body. Recent focus in the field of epigenetics has demonstrated it is possible to alter genetic expression by modifying the activation of certain genes, switching them on or off, without altering gene sequences (instruction sets) themselves. Changes in various environmental or external influencers such as nutrition, hormones, or exposure to toxins can result in a corresponding change in genetic expression.

Re-encoding is about activating special parts of our DNA so as to provide new and enhanced information to our DNA instruction sets. It is about altering, or re-encoding, the gene sequences on our DNA strands based on this information. As will be expounded upon in detail throughout the book, this is achieved by activating memory held within a specific part of our DNA, which is separate from the instruction sets, that helps the DNA instructions and our bodies remember how to operate efficiently and effectively. Re-encoding involves enhancing communication between these two parts of our DNA—the memory, which holds information, and the instruction sets, which govern our chemistry and biological response.

> Re-encoding is about activating special parts of our DNA so as to provide new and enhanced information to our DNA instruction sets. It is about altering, or re-encoding, the gene sequences on our DNA strands based on this information.

To some, this might seem inconceivable or impossible, but given the evidence and the mechanism by which this occurred, it is difficult to deny that it is indeed possible. I, myself, was often stunned and amazed at the explanations I received. I frequently grappled with the dilemma of how I could provide proof and solid evidence that would verify and provide credibility to the information I was gathering and my understanding of what was happening to me. Most often, I had very little prior knowledge (and therefore little bias) on a subject when conducting these inquiries and had no idea of the magnitude or profoundness of the answer to the questions I posed. Secondly, I had personal, firsthand experience. It was happening to me. The information received through these journeys and channels came from the etheric, which is a more universal source and a limitless source of knowledge. Therefore, the information in my mind is likely to be less intellectually constrained or biased than any scientific theory might be, as long as objectivity can be maintained and the message is not misconstrued. This unique method of information gathering, I would suggest, lends itself to the authenticity and validity of the message presented in this book.

The specificity and nature of my symptoms, along with the diagnoses, provided a corollary for what was being explained to me. I subsequently used scientific theory and the existing work of others to explain and verify the information provided to me. Many of the resources I came across in the aftermath of my inquiries and those that are quoted in this book provide proof that the information is indeed correct, to the extent that information on the subject exists and has been written about today. I am not a scientist, a medical doctor, or an expert in the subject matter of some areas that I expound upon, particularly those involving complicated quantum physics and physiology, but I have done my best to preserve the integrity and accuracy of all sources of information that are included. I have endeavored to ensure that I have not taken the ideas and concepts out of context or misrepresented the authors. In a few cases, some of the explanations provided may be simplistic summaries of very complicated scientific and medical information, but I believe sufficient detail has been provided to help the reader understand the meaning in a way that serves the message and intent of this book.

This book is, therefore, a melding of visible and invisible, from existing information and documented evidence as well as from etheric knowledge sources that may be entirely new, creating a much more complete picture of the role of our true genetic inheritance and our DNA in disease. My journey demonstrates that medical science and biology cannot be separated from the more nonphysical, quantum aspects of who we are as biological organisms if we are to expand the boundaries of our current understanding about disease and how it can be addressed. It challenges currently held beliefs and ideas as well as incomplete theories about our genetics that cannot be fully explained by what science knows today. There are a lot of theories—scientific, esoteric, and spiritual—that suggest what *might* be possible in terms of genetic alteration and the eradication of disease. Some of this theory has been proven in controlled laboratory experiments. Real-life cases and stories as well as anecdotal evidence exist that also support these ideas and concepts. However, to my knowledge, nothing has been definitively explained or proven. It is readily apparent that conventional medical science largely excludes the notion of the involvement of nonphysical influences on disease, perhaps out of ignorance or owing to a lack of knowledge or evidence. In addition, more traditional and holistic approaches that focus on the energetic or mind-body-spirit aspects have similarly failed to fully explain the relationship of these energetic phenomenon on our physical body at the level of our cells and genes. This book is an integration of these two disciplines that, when combined with the intangible and tangible evidence from my own authentic and personal experience that goes beyond them both, results in a demonstration of what *is* possible.

If I began this book by claiming that it is possible to re-encode our genes, improve health outcomes, and potentially eliminate serious disease, based on everything that science knows so far and what is common belief about genetics, some of its readers would dismiss this text entirely. Others might continue to read, but with only an idle curiosity or a good dose of skepticism. After all, given our understanding of our three-dimensional reality that is based on knowledge advanced by science, we have no evidence (yet) that this is possible or any real idea of how this could possibly occur. (Note that for the purposes of the book, I refer to our current reality as being three-dimensional for simplicity's sake and understanding, although depending on the definition and source, it may also be considered four- and even five-dimensional.) Technological advancements in medical science and biology have enabled us to understand a great deal about our biological genes and the part that we can identify and measure, but still little about the remaining portion that to date we cannot. Although the exact nature and function of this other part is unknown and somewhat mysterious, most have only examined the human genome within the context of current theories and within the confines of the laws of science that exist today. It is human nature and our cultural conditioning that encourages us to accept that science and our physicality hold all the answers. We are led to believe that existing and emerging theories are supported by evidence in all cases and we are rarely driven to look deeper.

Given the severity of my health conditions and disease over many years, I was not satisfied with the vague and often inconclusive explanations my doctors provided about what was happening to me and what the future held for me. I was not going to concede defeat when it seemed clear to me that my genes were controlling things in my body and the quality of my life. They were, by all accounts, dictating to some degree whether I lived, how well I lived, or if I died. Yet, I found it ironic that the mechanisms by which many of the physical therapeutic and pharmacological solutions currently offered for symptom relief and healing are not fully understood by medical science nor supported by evidence. My question was this: If we were able to develop a nonphysical means of influencing our genes to promote healing and the eradication of disease, would we dismiss this as a viable treatment option, even if we could not understand or measure the mechanisms by which it operated? It seemed no less risky to me given that neither approach necessarily could be fully supported by substantive physical evidence or a completely plausible explanation, given what we know today.

Mainstream, allopathic medicine approaches are predicated on the assumption that the answers lie in the physical body, regardless of its interaction with anything outside itself. The focus on what is happening in the physical body and the lack of recognition of the impact of external factors leads us further and further away from the truth of who we are as a human species. Focus on the physical aspects of ourselves has disconnected us from the capabilities that are inherent in us to self-regulate and self-heal, just as other living organisms in our universe are designed to do. In this way, we have become separate from the organizing forces and mechanisms that are at our disposal to guide our development, function, and ultimately our health. As Dr. Larry Malerba points out,

> body, mind, emotions, and spirit are inextricably united with the physical and social environment as one whole and cannot be divided except as an exercise of the mind. . . . Physical medicine rarely takes into account the deeper nature of the human being. Even when it does, it lacks an adequate framework to understand how these con-

nections create a whole, and consequently how to deal with them. … Conventional medicine prefers to limit its scope almost exclusively to the physical and because of this often ignores emotional triggers, psychological factors, and relationships. The blinders of medical science impose conceptual and perceptual limitations that result in a tendency for the profession to squeeze the round pegs of psychological and spiritual factors into the preconceived square holes of physical medicine.[4]

In order to find the answers to what our genetics are really all about and how we can work with them in achieving health and wellness, it is necessary to deconstruct this fundamental bias toward the physical body and accept that emotional, mental, spiritual, and environmental factors in our lives do exert an impact on our genetics. This is more than a vague notion about their influence in my mind—they have a significant and profound impact. I suggest, as some others do, that we simply cannot understand our genetics and their role in our health without due consideration of these factors. As I will demonstrate, these factors are by their nature all connected and cannot be viewed in isolation or manipulated individually without impacting each other and a person as a whole. Therefore, if we refuse to move beyond the limitations that are imposed on our understanding of genetics by focusing on the physical aspects of our genes and the portion of the chromosome we can identify and measure, we remain stuck in the perception that it is our biological genes that are in control of the chemical and biological responses in our bodies and, therefore, the main cause of disease, besides environmental influences. If we continue with this one-sided perspective, we will miss the point entirely—as well as the many opportunities for healing that a more expanded understanding may bring.

More recently, integrative approaches to medicine have begun to acknowledge the impact that energy in a general sense, regardless of a common understanding of exactly what this is, has on us at the level of the physical body. There is now a much greater appreciation for the interaction of more subtle forms of energy and the body that, to the vast majority, cannot be seen or currently measured. Many hold testament to the fact that its effects are recognizable and tangible. Traditional and holistic forms of energy medicine have been employed successfully by various cultures and peoples around the world for thousands of years. However, in modern medicine, "there is a peculiarly striking poverty of thought when it comes to the therapeutic application of energy, in spite of the education of all scientists regarding its nature and properties as formulated by physics. Science acknowledges the vital role of energy in the functioning of all life, but medicine acts as if it would constitute hocus-pocus to use energy as a healing modality."[5] The fact that many ancient ways of healing are the progenitors of techniques used today seems to be largely ignored. Ironically, medical diagnostic testing devices such as MRIs, CT scans, ECGs, or the machines used in radiation therapy use energy to detect certain conditions or ailments and to affect the energetic state of the body as a form of treatment.

Fortunately, more and more research as well as evidence is coming to the fore that is based on these putative (unmeasurable) interactions involving energy, providing answers about our genetics that medical science may have previously been unreceptive to. The human body more recently has been described as a "physical containment vessel," designed as "an energetic relay station, and a vehicle designed to receive and transmit a wide array of wave forms, vibrations, electromagnetic phenomena, and psychic and spiritual energies."[6] We are beginning to weave together a more complete picture of the physical body and the mechanisms of disease by integrating our knowledge of physiology, psychology, biology, quantum physics, and consciousness. But no one, to my knowledge, has proposed a single, popularly accepted model or view of exactly how this works.

So, what if we expand our notion of reality a little further to include these unmeasurable aspects of energy, which could perhaps change the current and popular position on the nature of our genetics entirely? What if we examine these aspects to answer questions such as: What happens when the body is exposed to higher vibrational or electro-magnetic energies? Where do these energies come from, how are they organized, and exactly what is contained in these energies that seems to impact our bodies in such profound ways? Can we access and utilize them to affect healing and potential change at the cellular and genetic level in our own physical bodies? What is it about us that might make us conducive to these changes? My personal journey did exactly that, and it led me to some profound and critical discoveries about our genetics that answer these questions. Through personal experience and unique sources of knowledge as well as scientific evidence, I am able to demonstrate why and how these answers can be supported. It is intended as a personal testament to the extraordinary capabilities we have in shaping our health by altering our DNA through our own conscious awareness.

In the first few chapters, the book provides a foundation around the basic principles of quantum (multidimensional) fields and quantum dynamics, upon which subsequent ideas and concepts about the nature of disease and genetics are built. To some, this might seem extraordinarily detailed and onerous, but without it, it may be impossible to grasp the ideas that are promoted throughout the remainder of the book as being perfectly reasonable and logical. To medical experts and practitioners, the skeptics and the undecided, these chapters represent an opportunity to see what is presented in this book as being founded in scientific evidence and existing theory, as opposed to unsubstantiated esoteric, spiritual supposition or rhetoric. Understanding our quantum nature, as a scientific as well as an etheric phenomenon, is critical to developing an appreciation for the astounding power that nonphysical influences in our energetic environment have over us as biological organisms and over our genetic fate. To my knowledge, the two have not been linked and fully explained. This understanding is essential for developing an ability to work with these influences to effect change at the cellular and DNA level and, ultimately, in creating the desired results with regard to re-encoding our genes to alter the information provided to our DNA. Later chapters summarizing scientific support for energetic mechanisms at the cellular and genetic level are also complicated and include some medical terminology. Thus, in order to facilitate comprehension of the concepts presented in this book, many are repeated and reiterated as reminders of their fundamental importance throughout.

There may be some readers who will be more interested in the story and the circumstances that surround my case. Sufficient detail and justification has been provided to give credibility to the enormity of the changes I personally experienced and document here, and so instead of making unsubstantiated claims, I have provided supporting evidence through a description of improvements in my health status wherever possible. Others may want to focus on learning about the consciousness tools that can be employed to work toward this ultimate objective. The tools described much later in the book involve working with conscious intent, which requires, at minimum, an understanding of quantum concepts at a basic level. It is difficult to develop appropriate and effective intentions in these exercises if we do not know what we are asking for and why.

Therefore, the reader may find it helpful to return to the fundamental concepts highlighted throughout the book from time to time to make sense of what has been written in subsequent chapters, particularly if the first pass is insufficient. Readers—whether practitioners, patients, scientific or spiritual enthusiasts—are encouraged to strive as much as possible to grasp some of the more technical and in-depth knowledge provided. For within this message lies the key that each of us holds to understanding the mechanism of disease and for working with the tools to unlock humanity's potential in manifesting health and wellness by re-encoding our genes through new information provided to our DNA.

1

The Demise of My Health

I myself have wounded myself in the journey
I am myself an obstruction in my own path

My home is becoming more and more distant
I have been walking backwards

Perhaps my destination is inside me.

KHALID SOHAIL, "SAFAR"[1]

Many of us come into this world seemingly perfect, and I suppose I was no different in that regard, having arrived as a baby of over eight pounds in the late 1950s, born into a very average Canadian family. During my childhood years, I was reasonably healthy, had an excellent diet, was involved in many extracurricular activities, and got plenty of exercise. In my twenties, thirties, and early forties, I was a very avid runner, mountain climber, and biker as well as skier and hiker. I received two postsecondary degrees and had a successful career. Well adjusted, you might say, in every regard. Nothing in my family medical history stood out as being extraordinary: three of my grandparents had died from cancer, one of them had a severe form of arthritis, my father had survived an aortic aneurism, and my mother and siblings had some thyroid issues. In the absence of any major diseases or medical conditions of my own or my immediate family members until I was almost fifty, I assumed this was all par for the course and that I came from perfectly good genetic stock.

It is quite common for people to dismissively remark upon being diagnosed or stricken with a disease or medical condition that "it runs in the family." Even in the absence of genetic testing or the appearance of symptoms or the disease itself, some simply resign themselves to the fact that they will most certainly succumb to it in the future, as if it were a fait accompli. After all, they say, "it's genetic." Many appear to have concluded that aside from disease and symptom management strategies, whether allopathic or holistic, there's nothing we can do to change our genetics. It seems we have actually accepted a less-than-perfect genetic state as the status quo. We assume that this is how human evolutionary biology works. This attitude has become deeply engrained in us, and our silent response to this issue indicates that we have condoned this approach to our health.

After a long period of doing what I thought were all the right things to maintain a healthy lifestyle, things started to change. My health began to deteriorate significantly over the course of six years. Although I did not realize it at the time, in reality, my decline and disease processes had begun a long time before that, well masked by my self-perceived healthiness, fitness level, and tenacity, as well as my lack of self-awareness. What ensued was an unraveling of my genetics, literally. I fell apart. Eventually, I became a genetic casualty, and it was apparent that I clearly was not as perfect as I had once thought.

Over the years, I had experienced a few accidents, including a bad rock-climbing fall impacting my low back and sacroiliac (SI) joints; a number of herniated discs in my neck, middle, and lower back from both gym and car accidents; as well as several mountain-bike accidents. None of these had left me seriously incapacitated or dysfunctional, and

I chalked them all up to being part of the risk associated with more adventurous sports—weekend warrior wounds. When my professional career was going full tilt, I gradually began to experience significant pain and discomfort in my middle and lower back, sacroiliac joints, and hips. The middle-back problem turned out to be a rare, noncancerous tumor that occupied 85 percent of one of the vertebra in my thoracic spine. I underwent a month-long course of radiation therapy—the same treatment a cancer patient would have received in order to eradicate the tumor.

But, the pain following the radiation therapy never disappeared, becoming more pervasive, and despite an immense amount of investigation, including all sorts of diagnostic testing and imaging as well as therapy offered by the medical system, my doctors were unable to arrive at a definitive conclusion as to the real source of my malaise. After spending in excess of $75,000 in addition to the benefit coverage I received from two health care plans for diagnostics and therapy, I was no further ahead and nothing was providing relief. I turned toward holistic approaches to complement my existing treatment regimens. Further testing to determine possible sources of my ill health at that time subsequently revealed toxic heavy metals and organic substances, which, unbeknownst to me, I had contracted some seventeen years earlier while working as a laboratory technician, specializing in heavy metal analysis of petroleum samples. Then, through the process of intuitive inquiry, I discovered that I had a cancerous tumor on the right side of my jaw, close to the temporomandibular joint (TMJ). This was subsequently verified by several very skilled and gifted medical intuitives and health practitioners. Radiation treatment was not possible since I had already received the maximum allowable lifetime dose of radiation in dealing with the tumor on my thoracic spine.

I wanted to get well, and so I began to read voraciously; I meditated; I shed layer upon layer of my past and worked on uncovering aspects of myself that I had lost and forgotten along the way, examining every last inch of who I was right down to the soul level. I explored the neuro-physiology of pain from an energetic perspective. In my better moments, through some very deep sound and breath work, I had even managed to transcend some of the pain. However, even with the understanding I had recently gained about disease, its root causes, and the true nature of healing, my condition did not improve.

Then, through these same methods of detection, breast cancer was added to my ever growing list of diseases. My body systems were already taxed from the toxicity, and so chemotherapy did not seem like a safe or viable option for me. By that point, I had already gone through multiple rounds of prolotherapy, botox, and nerve-block injections, radiofrequency nerve ablations, chiropractic and acupuncture treatments, as well as a whole host of other physical and exercise therapies. I had covered an immense amount of ground during this time, exploring a vast array of healing modalities including body energy work, traditional Chinese Five Element energy medicine, Shamanic and indigenous healing methods, and two techniques focused on soul and spiritual energy clearing. While they had been instrumental in my healing thus far, and had likely pulled me back from the brink on a few occasions, they had failed to address my symptoms, physiological dysfunction, and disease in any significant way. Although I certainly could see how some of the toxic exposure and injury issues had pushed me over the edge, I was convinced there had to be an underlying cause for all of this. Or was it simply my genetics?

Regardless, as is my nature, I pushed even harder and tried to become a little more active after so much downtime. Not even a month after a brief attempt at some very modest cycling, I had another accident, this time completely separating my right shoulder, tearing both of the main supporting ligaments. After a lengthy wait for surgery, and even after the surgical repair itself, things showed little improvement. During the course of my postsurgical monitoring, when I continued to complain about my unresolved condition, much to my surprise, diagnostic imaging revealed that my cervical spine was damaged and was now self-fusing, along with areas of my thoracic and lumbar spine. This was consistent with the images taken over the last seven years that had shown progressive signs of spinal degeneration. When coupled with my history, I now realized this was probably due to an uncontrolled inflammatory condition that went undiagnosed and untreated for many years. Prolonged, chronic inflammation can affect the axial skeleton, ligaments, and joints—most notably, the spine and sacroiliac joints. The inflammation produces chemicals that damage the bone and eat away at the cartilage between the bones, so the body tries to repair the damage, with scar tissue and new bone tissue, and heal the bone by depositing calcium around the area of damage, eventually causing the spine to fuse.

I was referred to a doctor who specializes in functional medicine. Functional medicine utilizes a holistic and integrated approach that examines the interrelationship of genetics, the environment, and lifestyle factors that can influence long-term health and chronic disease states. From the functional perspective, I surmised, there had to be an underlying cause for my symptoms and disease. We did genetic testing on all twenty-three of my chromosomes, which revealed a number of mutations associated with cancer, chronic inflammation, and my body's inability to detoxify, among others.

My understanding at that time was that genetic mutations (variations) were really just an indication of propensity of a person's predisposition toward expressing a trait, a disease, or a medical condition. Just because someone has genetic mutations, it does not mean that they will be expressed or will actually manifest as disease. Although my genetic testing results did seem to confirm the likelihood of the various diseases and dysfunction, they still did not explain the exact mechanism, the ultimate source of them, or why I did not improve with physical intervention and treatment. Epigenetics is a field of medicine that is based on the premise that it is the environment that dictates whether or not those particular genes are expressed. The environmental triggers that had played out in the manifestation of my diseases definitely seemed to be injury, exposure to toxins, and radiation, which may have contributed to the damage to my DNA and the mutations reported in my genetic testing results.

As I searched for answers and became more learned on the subject of DNA, I started to expand my definition of *environment*. Further reading and explorations into the nonordinary, cosmic realms, primarily via personal channeling and healing sessions, yielded some astonishing and vital clues. It became apparent to me, as has been proposed by others, that science currently only explains a portion of our genetics. New evidence, as well as the information that was presented to me, suggests that the remainder of the DNA is actually nonphysical in nature and, although of seemingly intangible origins, nevertheless has an astoundingly significant influence on who we are and what we actually manifest in terms of our health and well-being. Slowly, over the course of a year, I put the pieces together, corroborating my own experience and medical diagnostic evidence with the work of those who are pioneering new research and theories in this emerging field. I began to see how the invisible factors that science currently does not measure (yet are so apparent to those more versed in navigating and operating in these realms) had created an appropriate energetic milieu—a mosaic of emotional, mental, and spiritual factors that had as much, if not more, influence on creating the state of poor health that had become my reality.

I began to realize that DNA defines every aspect of who we are, right down to the cellular level, and stipulates how we respond to the information that is provided to us as biological organisms. Fortunately, under the right conditions, the body and our cells have the capacity to self-diagnose, repair, and regulate in order to heal and to maintain a healthy, balanced state. This is how nature designed us and other living organisms. Deeply engrained cultural behaviors and beliefs have led many to hold firmly to the ideal that health is only about physical symptom relief, as opposed to true healing. Healing, in my experience, is about addressing the emotional, mental, and spiritual factors and the DNA that they impact. It is about activating dormant and hidden aspects of ourselves and our DNA with our consciousness to essentially turn on these natural healing mechanisms. What I discovered was that it is our DNA, but not just our biological DNA, that is the biggest contributor to disease, as I will go on to demonstrate. The healing process may or may not require some physical intervention or support provided to the body to help facilitate natural healing mechanisms that the changes in our DNA are meant to invoke. Diet, supplementation, and some supportive therapies and treatments, such as acupuncture, massage, IV therapy or injections, detoxification protocols, and even exercise, may be helpful for some. It is important to remember that as complex, multidimensional beings, changes may be influenced and apparent at any and all levels—physical and nonphysical.

> **“**
> **Healing, in my experience, is about addressing the emotional, mental, and spiritual factors and the DNA that they impact. It is about activating dormant and hidden aspects of ourselves and our DNA with our consciousness to essentially turn on these natural healing mechanisms. 🟦🟦**

What follows is an attempt to explain this more complete version of what DNA really is—how it influences our cells and genetic response as relates to disease. I describe the means by which we can alter our own DNA to effect positive changes in our health by re-encoding our genes. It is not necessary to be a healing practitioner, an intuitive, or a cellular or genetic expert. Some defer the responsibility for their health to the knowledge and expertise of others, expecting professionals to know or to do something to them to heal them or to improve their condition. In actual fact, as my case suggests, it is possible to effect change in the state of one's own health (and DNA), without significant physical intervention, a definitive diagnosis, or external support, by way of the methods described in this book. Regardless of the approach, whether undertaken alone or when the assistance of others is sought for complementary or supporting therapy or treatment, the responsibility for change rests firmly with the patient. The practitioner facilitates the potential for healing, not the healing event itself. Therefore success, in my mind, can only be achieved when this important differentiation is understood and embraced by the patient along with a genuine desire to heal.

Given today's understanding of DNA, some have surmised that in theory it must be possible to alter the genome by some physical or chemical means. There is also a substantial amount of information available on how we can influence our genetic expression. However, I have gone one step further in explaining how we can actually re-encode our genes, why this is possible, and the mechanism by which this can be done. By working within our own capabilities, we possess the opportunity to create a different state of health in our bodies through self-regulation and self-healing. We can actually become more of the perfect person that we were intended to be.

2

The Truth about
Our DNA

Intelligent and Unmeasurable
Fields of Influence

You are your body; the body that you can see and touch is only a thin illusory veil. Underneath it lies the invisible inner body, the doorway into Being, into Life Unmanifested. Through the inner body you are inseparably connected to this unmanifested One Life . . .

ECKHART TOLLE[1]

THE DNA WE CAN MEASURE

The generally accepted view of conventional human genetics is that we have twenty-three pairs of chromosomes, each chromosome containing hundreds to thousands of genes. Our chromosomes are long strands of DNA (deoxyribonucleic acid) molecules that contain many genes, each with specific gene code sequences to synthesize structural and regulator proteins that ultimately define who we are in terms of our physical

21

structure and biological function, along with all of our inherited traits, conditions, and behaviors. As a result, DNA is like a fingerprint and is unique to each person. The instructions and job orders necessary for human development, function, and our biological inheritance are governed by our DNA, which oversees the roughly seventy to one hundred trillion cells in our bodies.

According to almost all mainstream scientific sources, DNA molecules consist of two biopolymer strands coiled around each other to form a double-helix shaped structure that looks much like a twisted ladder. These two DNA strands are linked by pairs of nucleobases, commonly known as *bases*. The four bases are guanine (G), adenine (A), thymine (T), and cytosine (C), which are joined together in a chain of bonds, much like the rungs of a ladder, connecting the two strands of the helix. The structure conforms to what is referred to as *base pairing rules* in which only certain bases are combined under normal conditions (A with T, and C with G).[2] It is the coding sequence or order of these four bases that carries the genetic information that facilitates biological assembly, function, and reproduction.

DNA is found mainly in the cell nucleus. Another type of nucleic acid known as RNA (ribonucleic acid) is common in the cytoplasm, the liquid material inside the cell and outside of the nucleus. Watson and Crick, the scientists responsible for discovering the structure of DNA, indicate that the RNA copies the DNA message in the nucleus and carries it out to the cytoplasm where, at the location of a subcellular organelle called a ribosome, proteins are made based on the genetic code. In addition, several types of RNA are involved in the utilization of genetic information. In the nucleus, the DNA code is transcribed or copied into a messenger RNA (mRNA) molecule. In the cytoplasm, the mRNA code is translated into amino acids. Translation is orchestrated at the ribosome, where transfer RNA (tRNA) reads the genetic code and selects the appropriate amino acids to add to growing proteins.[3]

There are literally hundreds of thousands of chemical reactions occurring in a given cell per second, and these are occurring simultaneously and in unison in each cell of the body. Being the complex biological organisms that we are, one would assume that in order to orchestrate the myriad of biological functions that take place within us, some of which are highly specialized, we must have a large number of coding genes to serve this purpose. This must also require a sophisticated communication system to carry out these vital functions with precision, impeccable coordination, and timing.

The Human Genome Project, launched in 1990 to map the entire human genome, found instead that there were far fewer of these than expected, somewhere on the order of about twenty thousand to twenty-five thousand. When this was discovered, it seemed inconceivable to some that such a small portion of our physical DNA, less than 5 percent of the chromosome, could realistically hold the entire DNA blueprint governing all aspects of our biological development and function. While it has been proven that the coded portion of our genes accounts for our biologically inherited traits such as the color of our hair and eyes, as well as other physical features such as height, what about the rest? If each cell contains the same blueprint, how do cells acquire the different appearances and functions owed to variations in genetic expression?

Science tells us that every cell in the body has the same genes, all with the same potential—but what distinguishes one cell from another and what genes get expressed? Stem cells, which are a kind of undifferentiated cells capable of giving rise to other cells, use the genetic information and have the potential to become any cell type, a blood cell or a kidney cell for example, depending on what molecular environment they are placed in. "Each normal cell has the ability to control certain messages or codes to be opened and translated, while others are set aside and ignored. In other words, cells prevent certain genetic messages from being expressed."[4] But the question remains, what tells the cell to turn off a message or express it? We know that genes are passive, and they do not do anything unless they are acted upon by something else. Science has not come up with a definitive answer to this fundamental dilemma. What the Human Genome Project seems to suggest is that the conventional, linear, three-dimensional interpretation of our biological genes does not seem to explain all of our biological functioning.[5]

A more recent international project called ENCODE (the Encyclopedia of DNA Elements) has moved away from describing the genome and toward providing more detailed information on what the genome actually does. The project's goal is to catalog every nucleotide within the genome that does something, including the non-encoding portion, which scientists admit is functional but yet to be fully understood. This attempt has generated some criticism within the medical and scientific communities, with some claiming that it has generated very little new information of physiological or evolutionary importance from this detailed library of "genomic parts data." The project has also stirred up a considerable amount of debate around how much of the DNA needs to be encoded to impact or cause disease, relative to the nonencoded portion. The ENCODE project has mapped all of the known genetic variants (known as single nucleotide polymorphisms or SNPs) and correlated these to various diseases. What researchers found was that just 12 percent of the SNPs responsible for them lie within the protein-coding areas. They also showed that compared to random SNPs, the disease-associated SNPs are more likely to lie within functional, noncoding regions of the genome.[6]

Neither do our genes explain the ultimate source of disease when you consider that "defective genes acting alone only account for about 2 percent of our total disease load," says Bruce Lipton, author of *Biology of Belief*.[7] For example, he says that 95 percent of breast cancers are not due to inherited genes and that many malignancies in a significant number of cancer patients are due to environmentally induced epigenetic alterations and not defective genes.[8] Epigenetics describes the function of epigenomes, which are chemicals and switches on our DNA that tell the genes how to operate and when to turn on or off. Although science has linked many genes to different diseases and traits, these are not activated until something triggers them. He emphasizes that we've become so engrained in our culture to believe that genes control biology that we've actually forgotten a single important truth: "When a gene product is needed, a signal from its environment, not an emergent property of the gene itself, activates expression of that gene."[9] Environmental factors can, in fact, rearrange gene sequencing creating genetic mutations.[10]

Technically speaking, genes themselves, and genetic variations in particular, are not responsible for creating disease. "We do not inherit a disease state per se. Instead, we inherit a set of susceptibility factors to certain effects of environmental factors and, therefore, inherit a higher risk for certain diseases."[11] Our genetic code, or genotype, is expressed in response to our external environment and our experience of a particular environment, which includes lifestyle factors such as diet, alcohol consumption, exercise, beliefs, thoughts, and emotions, as well as physical factors such as injury, toxicity, and immunity. These environmental factors alter the way our genes are expressed, and this is referred to as a *phenotype,* which is essentially another term for disease. Obviously, not all of our genes are expressed at any one time, nor will a particular code result in the same expression every time.

The question, however, remains: Is the physical environment as we currently understand it sufficiently able to explain inheritance and disease fully? Are all of the instructions coming from this environment? The quest for answers by mainstream science has been focused largely on clues from the physical world and what can actually be observed and measured. Mechanisms associated with the nonfunctional, nonencoded portion of the DNA molecule or those by which we interact and experience our physical world have largely been ignored. Therefore, what if we expanded the notion regarding the sphere of influence that might be impacting our DNA to include more than just our physical environment? Is it possible that the remaining 95 percent of the noncoding portion of our chromosome that scientists used to commonly refer to as "junk DNA" is involved in a nonphysical way that we might not expect? My personal experience and research ascertains that this is most definitely the case.

QUANTUM INFLUENCERS OF DNA

Fields of Influence

Despite the intensive study that has ensued regarding the human genome, it remains clear from what has been established and is measurable thus far that the complexities of the human body cannot reasonably be orchestrated by our biological DNA alone. As a result, the idea that there may be nonphysical, off-body influences on the genome now becomes more plausible. The concept of fields begins to set the stage for the development of an alternate view on how our genes might actually work. It lends itself to the possibility that the information our DNA uses to instruct the body to carry out its functions may be stored at a nonlocal level, away from the physical location of the chromosome in the body. A *field* is defined as "a matrix or medium which connects two or more points in space, usually via a force, such as light, gravity, or electromagnetism. The force is usually represented by ripples in the field or waves." More aptly put, it is a region of influence.[12] A field then, is essentially an integrated, invisible system consisting of energy or matter.

In the truest sense, we know that energy is a form of information. Despite the fact that fields are generally invisible, science has proven the existence and effects of some fields because they are actually *veritable,* or measurable. These include those that affect the human body including electrical, magnetic, and acoustic fields. Other fields have been identified by science that are referred to as being *putative,* which means they cannot be seen, touched, or perceived directly, nor measured. L-fields and T-fields, which are electrical and thought fields, fall into this category. Many who work in the field of holistic and vibrational medicine interact with the human energy field, which is another example of a putative field. This is a field that is considered to be the medium through which external information is exchanged with the physical body, through various energy planes and energy structures (chakras) or pathways (meridians) that penetrate the physical body (as a form of dense energy or matter) and its immediate vicinity and regulate all body functions. The body itself also represents a field. In fact, Cyndi Dale, author of *Subtle Body,* says that "every cell in the body and every thought generates a field. Every energy body, meridian, and chakra pulses its own field. In total, the field emanating from your body alone would occupy more space—or more 'anti-space'—than your physical self. In many ways, you are your fields."[13]

On a larger scale, Albert Einstein believed that the universe is composed of interconnected force fields. Physicists have described some of these fields, "viewing them as constructs of finite reality held within a greater infinity. Because of these fields, reality is both local (or here and now), and nonlocal, which means that everything is interconnected."[14] Given the concept of fields, it is apparent that the physical body is not isolated or separated from these fields, but rather, an integral part of them and their influence. Dale suggests that

> human and personal biofields also interconnect with greater fields that work in two directions; they receive and draw energy from us and also provide energy to us. Because we are actually composed of fields—as is the world—we have to see ourselves as interconnected rather than self-sustaining, constantly involved in the flux of becoming something new even as we shape and reshape the world.[15]

Thus, the concept of fields and the interaction we have with them most definitely lends itself to the idea that there is an energetic information exchange between the fields that define us and our physical bodies, and those that are more external to us. These external fields contain temporally and spatially nonlocal, nonphysical information that conforms to the definition of something that is quantum in nature. The concept of nonlocality moves us beyond the paradigm of what Ervin Laszlo refers to as "local realism," which he says still dominates the modern world and science. This is the assumption that any phenomenon that we observe is deemed to be local, meaning physical effects propagate through space at a certain speed before they disappear with increasing distance. The reality assumption infers that all things that exist must have values or characteristics intrinsic to them that prove their existence, rather than them being created as a result of their relationship with one another or by their observation.[16] Nonlocality as a departure from this prevailing concept of local realism leads us to the next step in our logical progression in identifying the ultimate source of influence on our DNA.

Quantum Fields

An object exists in a specific location, but a quantum field does not since it is nonlocal and its components are everywhere. Therefore, a quantum field would theoretically penetrate the physical body at the deepest level, its cells, organs, and organ systems, and extend beyond it. These unique properties explain how organisms at any level in nature can be affected by their interactions with each other and their external environments, without being connected by some physically real medium.

> In the quantum world, quantum fields are not mediated by forces but by an exchange of energy, which is constantly redistributed in a dynamic pattern. This constant exchange is an intrinsic property of particles, so that even "real" particles are nothing more than a little knot of energy that briefly emerges and disappears back into the underlying field. According to the quantum field theory, the individual entity is transient and insubstantial. Particles cannot be separated from the empty space around them.[17]

The notion of "Morphic Fields" was first developed by Rupert Sheldrake as a means of explaining the function and behavior of natural biological organisms. He believes they are comparable to quantum fields in many respects as they share many of the same fundamental characteristics. He describes Morphic Fields as being nonlocal, like a quantum field, where "an effect is instantaneous and unaffected by distance. Morphic Fields contain nonphysical patterns of information that manifest effects in the physical state."[18] This invisible field is considered to be causal because it interacts with observable matter, organizing their form, development, and function. Within the body, for example, each organ has a Morphic Field, as does each tissue, cell, organelle, or molecule. There are nested hierarchies of fields within fields. On a larger scale, ecosystems, solar systems, and even galaxies have fields.

Sheldrake says that the Morphic Field is characterized by an inherent or natural vibration, known as a resonant frequency, that holds information about the system's potential form and behavior, which he describes as being analogous to genetic information. The information may actually be the memory of everything that has ever happened to a particular organism or entity, stored and communicated vibrationally. When the fields of two similar organisms interact with each other, the natural or resonant frequency of the one field induces the second field into vibrational motion until the two fields resonate with each other at the same frequency. This is known as *morphic resonance.* It is the mechanism by which Sheldrake believes information from one organism is stored and transmitted to the next, providing a possible explanation for inheritance. Thus, each organism's field attracts the system (a unit of the physical world characterized by unique, inherent vibration) and the information or instructions inherent in that system with which it is associated, toward its mature form, and it arouses behavior in that system. Therefore according to this theory, as an example, he surmises that the Morphic Field of the tadpole would encode the physical form and instinctive behavior of the mature frog.

Sheldrake explains that morphic resonance takes place on the basis of similarity, likely owing to comparable resonant frequencies that are associated with organisms of the same species or biological origins. He says that the tendency for an organism's field to resonate with a field containing information from its own past states is the most probable, because it is more similar to itself in the past, especially in the immediate past, than to any other organism. Information, however, is not only exchanged between a system and its field. Similar fields, by resonance, also influence similar systems. Thus, according to the Morphic Field hypothesis, living organisms "inherit not only genes, but also habits of development from past members of their own species."[19] Sheldrake suggests that

> the morphic influence of a past system might become present to a subsequent similar system . . . by passing "beyond" space-time and then "reentering" wherever and whenever a similar pattern of vibration appeared. Or it might be connected through other "dimensions." Or it might go through a space-time tunnel to emerge unchanged in the presence of a subsequent similar system.[20]

There is another field—called the Akashic Field—that offers an additional means of understanding what kind of information is stored in quantum fields and how this might influence our DNA. The notion of the existence of the Akashic Field is not new and originated in ancient Indian spiritual culture thousands of years ago. The Akashic Field has similarities to the Morphic Field and in many ways may very well be an extension of this concept. It is also considered to be quantum and multidimensional in nature and is viewed as "an all pervasive foundation that contains all knowledge of the human experience and the entire history of the universe."[21] This means that the Akashic Field is an *informed field* that holds information and, thus, enormous potential in influencing who we are as living organisms—our form, function, and behavior. It has been demonstrated that the Akashic Field can be accessed through expanded states of conscious awareness, such as those achieved through meditation or by other spiritual means. The precise nature and function of the Akashic Field as it relates to our DNA will be described in detail in subsequent chapters.

The *informed* quantum field concept as presented here presents a departure from the conventional understanding of genetics where physical DNA are seen as *generators* and the source of the information provided to the body for its development and function. Instead, in a quantum context, we can now view DNA more clearly as *receivers* of nonlocal, quantum information that ultimately governs the chemical reactions and biological responses in the body. Therefore, the DNA blueprint, as it is known, is stored and utilized within a quantum field as a dynamic energetic record, instead of in a physical state. Going forward, viewing the Akashic Field as a quantum field offers the most plausible explanation for the source and mechanism of influence on our genes that resides outside our physical bodies.

Therefore, the DNA blueprint, as it is known, is stored and utilized within a quantum field as a dynamic energetic record, instead of in a physical state.

It is important to point out, however, that while the concept of quantum fields as being the supplier of information appears to be substantiated, according to the information I have received, the prevailing theory that resonance is the mechanism of information transmission may not necessarily be correct, as I will go on to demonstrate.

Quantum Relationships

In order to explore the possible origins and nature of our genetic inheritance beyond its known biological source more fully, it is necessary to first examine the concept of quantum field dynamics in more detail. An exact and generally accepted definition of how quantum aspects explain our physical world, the interrelationship of all living things, as well as their behavior and precise function, has not been established by science, owing largely to their putative nature.

Relationships of entities in quantum fields appear to operate seamlessly and mysteriously by some kind of invisible, sentient quality or intelligence. This intelligence implies that somehow quantum information is transmitted, received, and interpreted in some way by its participants, who are an integral part of the field, to manifest a result—a kind of form or function. It is the results of the interactions of these relationships that are measurable by science, and that has led to the conclusion that "quantum-ness" can create change in both energetic and physical states. The concept of its intelligence also infers that it can communicate with us through a form of language, which is believed to occur outside the normal functioning of the brain. This language is consciousness.

Quantum-ness through its hallmark attributes—namely, coherence, nonlocality, and entanglement—can be used to describe life at the most fundamental level. Quanta, the smallest identifiable element of the quantum world, do not exist in a single place in any given moment, but instead, exist everywhere at once. Until they are observed or measured, quanta have no definite characteristics and can exist simultaneously in several states at once.[22]

Some of these quanta have matterlike properties, such as mass, gravitation, and inertia. Others have force-properties, making up the particles that convey effective interaction among matterlike quanta. Yet others have lightlike properties; they carry electromagnetic waves that include the visible spectrum. But none of the quanta are truly separate from one another, for—once having shared the same state—they remain interlinked no matter how far they may be from each other. And none behave as ordinary objects. They have both corpuscular and wave-properties, depending, it seems, on the way the experiments through which they are observed are set up. Moreover, when one of their properties is measured, the others become unavailable to observation and measurement.[23]

Quanta are in constant communication and interaction with each other, through the process of quantum nonlocality. They are connected or entangled with each other using information that is obtained by what is known as nonlocal quantum coherence.[24] The term *coherence* means that systems comprised of quanta exhibit a property by which any change in one of the parts of the system results in a change in all the others. These changes propagate through the system quasi-instantly and are enduring.[25] The importance of these quantum attributes lies in the fact that in isolation they are virtually meaningless. They can only be understood within the context of their relationships. Research also indicates that quanta, as the smallest identifiable units of matter, force, and light are not entirely separate realities, but rather, specific forms and bundles of underlying energy fields. We will examine these bundles of energy fields in more detail as other possible origins of genetic information are elaborated upon.

Quantum phenomenon are exhibited at all levels of life, whether at a microcosmic level (subatomic, DNA, cellular, organism, and the like) or macrocosmic level (universal or multidimensional). Thus, by quantum mechanisms, "atoms and molecules within organisms, and entire organisms and their environments, are nearly as 'entangled' with each other as microparticles that originate in the same quantum state."[26] This has important implications in understanding how quantum information can be transmitted to our DNA and our cells. Through quantum attributes, an organism can be in tune or coherent with nonlocal information. "The mutual entanglement of quanta indicates that information is subtly but effectively transmitted throughout the quantum world. As this informational linking is both instant and enduring, it appears to be independent of space as well as of time."[27] As Laszlo points out, this quantum coherence seems to be one of the only ways that explains how our atoms, molecules, and cells can respond instantaneously to the instructions they receive by making physical changes to themselves chemically or mechanically. No matter how diverse the cells, organs, and organ systems of the organism, they act as one.[28] "Through quantum effects, cells create a coherent field of information throughout the body. This 'biofield' supplements the ordinary flow of information with the multidimensional quasi-instant information needed to ensure the coordinated functioning of the whole organism."[29] When we look at the complexity in form and function of the human body and how things work together in such an intensely orchestrated and coordinated fashion, this makes sense.

Quantum Information Storage and Transmittal

The connected state that characterizes quantum fields means there is a relationship of everything to itself and to external realities, both locally and nonlocally through these fields. This is achieved through what is known as a *holographic property* in which the behavior of any part within a system can be organized by the whole because information is shared or represented at any and all levels in the system. A hologram represents the recorded pattern, or encoded information, created in this case when waves containing quantum information in a field interfere with each other. It is "a special type of wave interference pattern which takes two aspects of the same wave and recombines them to form a three-dimensional reality. A holographic system can carry a vast amount of information and every bit of information is contained everywhere in the hologram."[30] These quantum-type waves are coherent, nonlocal, and are entangled within the universe. The main holographic principle of the universe, that every part contains the whole—often described by the phrase, "As above, So below; As without, So within"—is thereby reflected in this view. In other words, what exists in the macrocosm also exists at the microcosm level. Physicists have described how the volume of a vacuum the size of a proton contains an energy density equivalent to all of the mass in the universe. This demonstrates the holographic concept that something as small as a subatomic particle can contain the imprint of the entire universe, and that there are many dimensional layers to the universe, where this infinite energy density is distributed.[31]

Therefore, "when something is holographic, any semblance of location breaks down . . . it is another way of saying that the information is distributed nonlocally."[32] The term *holofractal* is used to describe fractal or repetitive parts of this same hologram, represented at all levels of the universe and among living things. The information that is exchanged between levels—these levels being what is referred to as implicate order, meaning an *enfolded* or deeper level of reality at the nonlocal level, and an explicit order, meaning an *unfolded* or individual local level—is dynamic and in a state of continual flux and mutual reciprocation. By the holographic principle, neither we as organisms nor our cells or DNA can be separate from the holographic information contained at a nonlocal level. Therefore, we are interacting with more than the immediate environment that we perceive through our senses. We are constantly in contact with and exchanging this multidimensional information in a quantum manner. This principle also makes it possible for organisms to be a part of an undivided whole yet, at the same time, still possess their unique qualities.[33]

The Quantum Holography model attempts to explain the mechanism by which living organisms receive and process quantum, holographic information. Quantum Holography describes the universe as a self-organizing, interconnected, conscious, and holistic system. It explains how living organisms know what they know and how they utilize information. The theory, which has been validated experimentally, proposes that fluctuating quantum emissions, in the form of electromagnetic waves from any physical or material entity, carry information nonlocally about the "event history" of the quantum states of that entity. Quantum Holography fully describes everything about the states of the object that created it and is consistent with the principles of Morphic and Akashic Fields described earlier. The event history carried by the quantum hologram is an evolving record of every objective, subjective, and physical experience, in other words, its entire space-time history. The Quantum Holographic model prescribes that this history (quantum information) is stored in a wave interference pattern as a hologram.

These interference patterns from the emitted quanta carry an incredible amount of information, including the entire space-time history of that entity or person. Recent evidence has suggested that each of us has our own unique resonant, meaning natural and inherent, holographic memory and this memory is stored as an "image" or wave interference pattern, in what is called the "Zero Point Field." According to scientists, the Zero Point Field is defined as a nonlocal quantum realm that consists of "light that encompasses all of reality."[34] Although this field is in a near-vacuum state (which implies there is nothing in it), in actuality it is full of fluctuating emitting quantum particles in wave form, appearing and then disappearing from existence. The term "zero" in the Zero Point Field is used because fluctuations in the field are still detectable in temperatures of absolute zero, which is the lowest possible energy state where all matter has been removed and nothing is theoretically left to create motion.[35] Due to its quantum nature, it is also described as being ubiquitous and nonlocal. It can never lose its intensity or coherence and is capable of storing unlimited quantities of information. Most importantly, "the Zero Point Field is a repository of all fields and all ground energy states and all virtual particles—a field of fields."[36]

"The existence of the Zero Point Field suggests that all matter in the universe is interconnected by waves, which are spread out through time and space and can carry on to infinity, tying one part of the universe to every other part."[37] Through the Zero Point Field, we are interconnected to a nonlocal reality that permeates the cosmos.[38] As alluded to earlier, waves and wave fields are encoders and carriers of quantum information, or event history, and when they interfere with each other, they essentially share their information with each other. The result of these interference patterns, which are being generated continually, is a constant and infinite storage of holographic information. From a vibrational perspective, each of us is in constant resonance with our own personal quantum hologram or wave pattern. The unique resonant frequency that characterizes each one of us individually and that comprises our personal hologram will "act as a fingerprint to identify our nonlocal information stored in this Zero Point Field. By this mechanism, the event history of all matter, including us, is continually broadcast nonlocally by coherent quantum emissions and stored in the quantum holograph. The history is received by all other matter and us, in the Zero Point Field through this process of information exchange."[39]

The Quantum Holographic model presents a very compelling explanation of how information that governs our physical DNA and our biological functioning might be stored nonlocally. It suggests that we interact with this field and have access to the information or event history about ourselves that is stored there. From this, we can also surmise that our personal quantum holograms contain information about our past existence, including event history regarding circumstances when were perfectly healthy, which we can interact with in a quantum way. This is critical to our understanding going forward as we explore the means by which this information can be accessed and modified to communicate new messages to our DNA to prompt repair and regenerating functions in the case of disease.

> **"**
> Our personal quantum holograms contain information about our past existence, including event history regarding circumstances when were perfectly healthy, which we can interact with in a quantum way. **"**

The Akashic Field

Ervin Laszlo has gone a step further in characterizing a quantum field of holographic information and has called this the Akashic Field, or "A field," mentioned earlier. He describes this field as being something far greater than the Zero Point Field just described and believes it possesses more transcendent or esoteric-like properties. The word *Akasha* originates in Sanskrit and Indian cultures, referring to an "all-encompassing medium that underlies all things and becomes all things" or "cosmic sky," analogous to our idea of space. The Akashic Field isn't so much a location but rather a compilation of energies or frequencies that are implicit with its existence. It is real but so subtle that it cannot be perceived until it becomes the many things that populate the physical world. We do not directly interact with the Akasha through our normal, ordinary multisensory perception, but can interact with it through various practices that allow us to achieve higher states of consciousness, including meditation.[40]

> According to the philosophers of India, the whole universe is composed of two materials, one they call Akasha [the other is prana or life force]. It is omnipresent, [an] all-penetrating existence. Everything that has form, everything that is the result of combination, is evolved out of this Akasha. It is the Akasha that becomes the air, that becomes the liquids, that becomes the solids; it is the Akasha that becomes the Sun, the Earth, the Moon, the stars, the comets; it is the Akasha that becomes the human body, the animal body, the plants, every form that we see, everything that can be sensed—everything that exists. It cannot be perceived, it is so subtle that it is beyond ordinary perception; it can only be seen when it has become gross, has taken form. At the beginning of creation there was only this Akasha . . .[41]

The Akasha "was believed to conserve the traces of everything that ever happened in space and in time. Akasha is the enduring memory of the cosmos: it is the 'Akashic Record.'"[42]

Obviously, from the description, it is clear that the Akashic Field is an information field, and it is purported to be the basis of all living things. Nikola Tesla, the renowned scientist, suggests that there is an original medium that fills space, which he compared to the Akasha.

According to Laszlo, Tesla wrote that "this original medium, a kind of force field, becomes matter when prana, cosmic energy, acts on it, and when the action ceases, matter vanishes and returns to Akasha. Since this medium fills all of space, everything that takes place in space can be referred to it."[43] It is considered to be a complex and fundamental medium that carries within it all other fields, including the electromagnetic and gravitational fields, along with the Zero Point Field. The Akasha is therefore the element that records, conserves, and conveys information.[44] The basis of all life is seen to originate from the quantum vacuum's energy, and all of the parts of any organism system or entity interact with it. As this interaction takes place, its history is inscribed as memory, as a hologram upon the Akasha, by the mechanism of wave interference described previously. Thus, as Ervin Laszlo describes it, "the Akashic field is a field of quantum holograms, a kind of superconducting cosmic medium." He says that the quantum holograms created by the waves emitted by objects, including us and all biological organisms, entangle throughout the field through space and time. This produces a sequence of interference patterns that ultimately create a "superhologram," which is the integration of all other holograms and carries the information on all things that exist.[45]

We can see how this model extends to the human level, where the event history of humanity and the individual—every interaction, every thought, emotion, or experience is recorded as a hologram upon the Akasha. Therefore, the quantum hologram is, essentially, the recording device of the event history or information at all levels of life, from the subatomic, the cellular and the DNA level, to the individual, all the way to humanity as a whole. When we interact with the memory and information contained in the Akashic Field, it is real. As Ervin Laszlo points out, "access to the Akashic field—the Akashic experience—is a genuine and indeed fundamental element of human experience: as Edgar Mitchell [the prominent ex-astronaut] suggests in his book, we should regard it not as our *sixth* sense, but as our *first*—it is actually our most basic sense."[46] As we will see, these quantum fields of information feature prominently in understanding what informs our DNA and our cells and the means by which this intelligence can be transmitted.

> **Therefore, the quantum hologram is, essentially, the recording device of the event history or information at all levels of life, from the subatomic, the cellular and the DNA level, to the individual, all the way to humanity as a whole.**

Quantum Fields and Consciousness

The link between the information that is stored holographically in the Akashic Field and our bodies is our consciousness. Apparently, there is a considerable amount of interest being generated in genetic science as it relates to quantum bioholography and its assertion that there is a distinct and important relationship between the universal energy field, genetic response, and consciousness, consistent with the message of this book.[47] In fact, consciousness is the means by which we interpret this quantum information. It is such an integral part of our existence that the role of consciousness in explaining the science of life has captured the interest of scientists, neuroscientists, psychologists, and philosophers and is evolving into an entirely new science. It is beginning to weave its influence into mathematical formulas, theorems, experiments, and the interpretation of evidence in even the purest forms of science. It is becoming more and more difficult to fully explain ourselves and our world without its involvement. Many maintain human consciousness may very well be the driver for our reality. The phenomenon known as the observer effect offers the idea that nothing exists as a "thing" independent of our perception of it. It implies that our reality and aspects of our physical universe may be open to influence in some way through the involvement of consciousness.[48] The term *consciousness* described in this book is meant as an awareness that is separate from normal processes occurring in the brain such as cognition. The brain is merely the organ that manifests consciousness, as a means of providing a quantum experience to us in a local way.

Stuart Hameroff, a professor of anesthesiology and psychology and director for the Center for Consciousness Studies, has some interesting theories on the various mechanisms of consciousness. He also supports the idea of the existence of a quantum field that makes up the structure of the universe as described. He agrees that it is holographic, repeating at different scales, and that it exhibits nonlocal effects. Hameroff says that consciousness, as awareness, is a fundamental property that is built into this quantum field. He believes that it is intrinsic to the universe and that the raw precursors of consciousness are omnipresent, although perhaps not as all-encompassing as some who believe that consciousness in and of itself is a field. Hameroff suggests that quantum processes in microtubules in our brains connect to this quantum field at some fundamental level, and this is what gives rise to experience or awareness.[49]

Most importantly, consciousness is what connects our experience to our bodies. Negative or dysfunctional thoughts and emotions that result from our experiences are an indication that we may have incorrectly interpreted quantum information. The Akashic Field stores event history, including universal and self-knowledge about our connection to All That Is, our origins and purpose in life, our true potential, our soul's lessons and history, and even information pertaining to our ability to self-regulate our bodies and heal. This information is constantly being broadcasted in a quantum manner to our DNA and our cells and has not changed, although we may have. Through our own consciousness, by various means that will be described, we have forgotten or misinterpreted the information being broadcast. This, ultimately, translates to consequences in the physical body and

> The Akashic Field stores event history, including universal and self-knowledge about our connection to All That Is, our origins and purpose in life, our true potential, our soul's lessons and history, and even information pertaining to our ability to self-regulate our bodies and heal.

has a great deal to do with the end result, our genetic coding and our health. Sadly, very few have retained the conscious awareness of this information that is so vital to our health and the reality that we manifest, with the exception of mainly indigenous cultures, holistic practitioners, and spiritualists, whose lives and practices reflect this fundamental truth. Instead, the modern scientific mind has "broken the universe down into an unending array of parts, particles and components, thus creating the illusion that all of these bits are isolated and separate entities."[50] When we experience emotions of fear, guilt, or anger, we experience corresponding chemical changes in our bodies. The body responds by producing chemicals and a host of other psychosomatic responses, including disease. Most of us, however, are not versed in a deeper relationship with our bodies through our consciousness. Few can accurately discern the presence or nature of a disease that might be present without relying on external sources of information such as a diagnosis inferred from a medical laboratory test or diagnostic imagery. This is ironic when we consider that the holographic information throughout and around our bodies is nonlocal and quantum and is available for us to access and use to our benefit in achieving and maintaining a state of health.

With some knowledge and training, however, it is possible to "tune in" or direct our own consciousness in order to access and use the information contained in the Akashic Field to effect change in our bodies. By virtue of the fact that universal information is stored holographically there, we literally have access to the same cosmic energies or morphogenetic forces that comprise all life in the universe. Experiments have verified that through consciousness and various psychological, parapsychological, and spiritual healing techniques, we are able to connect transpersonally, telepathically, or telesomatically to communicate with the minds of others as well as interact and produce effects in their bodies.[51] Biofeedback techniques have proven that consciousness can be used to control body functions such as temperature, heart rate, and respiration rate. These effects, real and measurable, have been repeatedly demonstrated and documented. Cultures and indigenous peoples have shown for thousands of years that through various ceremonies, rituals, and protocols involving meditative or altered states of consciousness, it is possible to access a wide range of nonlocal information to understand, relate, and respond to the world, to one another, and to heal the body.

Our consciousness and quantum multidimensionality is, therefore, the key to healing and the manifestation of our fullest expression as a human being. Some of the consciousness tools that I describe later on in the book are examples of the means by which this can be accomplished for the purposes of re-encoding our genes.

> **Our consciousness and quantum multidimensionality is, therefore, the key to healing and the manifestation of our fullest expression as a human being.**

Personal Quantum Fields—the Merkaba

The notion that the physical body is encapsulated in layers of energy, sometimes referred to as the subtle or energetic body, has been around for thousands of years, and has now become quite commonplace. Its general acceptance has been confirmed by the prevalence of a multitude of healing modalities and body therapies involving energy throughout history and that exist today. Although the subtle energy layers of the body are not visible to everyone, learned practitioners and those who have the ability to view them with their "inner sight" agree that they represent the greater part of our "body-being," comprising as much as ninety-nine times more area than the physical body. These subtle energies "support, shape, and animate the physical body, often displaying intelligence that transcend human knowing . . . it is hardly a new idea to suggest that subtle energies operate in tandem with the denser, 'congealed' energies of the material body."[52] This field of energy has been described by many as having both particle and wave characteristics, which are evidence of its quantum attributes. These characteristics remind us of our dynamic nature—our bodies are more or less a state of energy that is constantly changing and evolving in response to various stimuli, as opposed to a thing or a more solid entity. When we begin to appreciate this, it is easier to see ourselves not in terms of the duality of what is *me* or *not me* in the physical sense, but instead, that we are part of a continuum, a quantum energy field that is the central engine of our being and our consciousness.[53]

Each of us has our own unique energetic signature, which is a natural, inherent frequency at which we vibrate. This energy, or frequency, is represented by our "light body" or light pattern. Our light body extends out to the edge of our energetic bodies (those commonly identified as the etheric, mental, emotional, and spiritual energetic bodies) and is bounded by a structured matrix of light, referred to as the Merkaba. It resonates at a very high vibration. The *Merkaba* is a Hebrew word that means "to ride," which means that our body-being rides upon this foundation. There are numerous historical references to the Merkaba, primarily as an ascension vehicle that allows us to transcend the limitations of our physical, three-dimensional reality into dimensions beyond, when the mind, heart, body, and spirit are integrated into this primal pattern of light. It is described in the Bible and the Torah and by many religious cultures including Christian, Egyptian, and Jewish as well as by mystics around the world. The Merkaba is believed to be a multidimensional portal into higher levels of consciousness.

Our Merkaba is what separates the local personal quantum field that immediately surrounds us and our physical body from the universal Akashic Field that lies beyond. The light matrix that characterizes the Merkaba appears as a structured form in the shape of a double tetrahedron and is what allows us to tie what is quantum to our physical form. The Merkaba Field is believed to be very complex, both in form and function. Accordingly, Rupert Sheldrake's notion of nested Morphic Fields would mean that technically the Merkaba Field and the universal Akashic Field are not mutually exclusive of one other (as described here for simplicity's sake), but rather, they are entangled with one another in a quantum, nonlinear way.

THE DNA THAT CANNOT
BE MEASURED

It has been demonstrated experimentally that our physical DNA functions by mechanisms beyond those that are chemical. This was brought about by the discovery that "the body is surrounded by a field of light and that DNA responds to and interacts with the various electromagnetic frequencies found in this field."[54] The Russian scientist Vladimir Poponin conducted an experiment involving a single molecule of physical DNA and light in which he discovered the DNA had a quantum field around it. In this field, he observed that the light patterned itself into a wave and that there was information contained in this field.[55] Other theories also acknowledge the relationship between our physical DNA and a more external field of influence, as well as DNA's ability to store and transmit light, which we will return to later. Scientists often describe quantum fields as being filled with "potentials" since the activity and response of a quantum field is dynamic and is affected by many factors, including human consciousness.[56]

One's personal field, bounded by the Merkaba, contains our Akashic information stored holographically as quantum light emissions and, therefore, has quantum, nonlocal characteristics. This information influences our DNA and provides it with the necessary instructions with which to oversee and orchestrate the cellular function and gene response in our bodies. As will be described in subsequent chapters, the electromagnetic energies contained within this personal quantum field have an exceptionally powerful influence over how this information is received and interpreted by our DNA.

Science does not currently acknowledge the existence of this field, nor its influence on our genes, because it cannot be measured. However, the mere action of DNA in our bodies suggests it has a quantum influence, particularly since we observe DNA as being nonspecific and nonspecialized. In other words, DNA is not specific to one particular aspect of the body like our fingernails, hair, or an organ. Everyone possesses a unique quantum DNA blueprint, which is their personal quantum holographic information package, existing in every single cell and part of their body. This explains how DNA intelligence can be communicated instantaneously and simultaneously to orchestrate biological and cellular functioning, when governed by the mechanism of quantum entanglement described earlier. Its quantum "collective intelligence" or "single consciousness" implies a kind of unity or Oneness in energy. Therefore, DNA is not completely physical, operating in a linear manner according to the existing laws of biological science, which is perhaps why it has evaded measurement by the scientific community thus far. It is also quantum.

Our DNA also functions in a nonphysical way and is governed by the intelligence that exists within our personal quantum field. It derives quantum information as energy from this field through our consciousness, which in turn dictates how we interpret the DNA blueprint instructions that translate as our biological response at the cellular and genetic level. The information is communicated imperceptibly and silently in a way that informs us via the brain as the bridge for the reality we perceive. As I will demonstrate further, our thoughts, emotions, and behaviors are driven largely by the energy that resides in this field, not by some nebulous or random influence from our brains.

> **"**
> **Our DNA also functions in a nonphysical way and is governed by the intelligence that exists within our personal quantum field. It derives quantum information as energy from this field through our consciousness, which in turn dictates how we interpret the DNA blueprint instructions that translate as our biological response at the cellular and genetic level.**
> **"**

Clearly, DNA is far more than it has traditionally been viewed as. It is more than the instructions for building pieces of protein that produce biological responses in the physical body through chemistry that we know about and can measure. Instead, it has a quantum component as well. The double helix that we so commonly associate with DNA is a schematic representation, but not what DNA actually looks like in multidimensional or quantum form. Three-dimensional animations show DNA as a compilation of shapes and building blocks that clump around each other in complex ways. However, it is generally accepted by the vast majority of those with more progressive spiritual beliefs and experience that we actually have ten strands of multidimensional DNA in addition to the two strands of biological (chemical) DNA, characterized by the three-dimensional structure that science currently can see. These ten strands represent the non-encoded portion of the chromosome, which are the quantum and spiritual aspects of who we are. This portion of our DNA contains a whole multitude of energies, all organized in a nonlinear, nonphysical, multidimensional way. These energies describe our uniqueness and are a record of the memory of who we are as souls in each lifetime. This record includes our divine and biological origins, our karma, the blueprint for our energetic bodies, our soul's purpose and life lessons, our soul's records (Akashic Records), as well as additional aspects of ourselves, including our Innate Self and Higher Self, among other spiritual attributes.

> The 90 percent of DNA is a reflection of your spirituality. The Akashic Record, the Higher Self, that which you seek that you call a "portal to the other side," is there. In a quantum state, these things are not actually in the chemicals at all. Think of all those chemicals together as a bridge, somehow a pipeline, a portal or quantum pointer to everything. Instead of thinking in a linear way that there is a compartment or a box where your Higher Self is, think of a doorway. If you could go there and see the quantum state of it, you would enter into a pipeline that takes you to everything that is. So understand that this 3D/quantum chemical bridge is a sacred influencer of the genome, and it's very large, containing most of the information in the Human blueprint of life.[57]

This description suggests that our quantum DNA is actually the progenitor of our biological DNA and represents the ultimate origin of all information provided to the biological instruction sets contained within the protein-encoded portion of the chromosome.

This description suggests that our quantum DNA is actually the progenitor of our biological DNA and represents the ultimate origin of all information provided to the biological instruction sets contained within the protein-encoded portion of the chromosome.

3

Quantum and Biological DNA

The Basis for Gene Encoding

Our gene's encoding tool consists of both the encoded portion of the chromosome (the biological aspect of our DNA) as well as the nonencoded portion (the quantum aspect of our DNA) together.

QUANTUM ORIGINS
OF GENETIC INFORMATION

As I pondered the significance of the nature of quantum information fields and the relationship to our DNA, I began to conduct regular channeling sessions in a particular dimension of consciousness to which I have been granted access. I was interested in learning about the ultimate origin of our genetics in this more esoteric and etheric context, given this multidimensional, quantum attribute that comprises our DNA. It was explained to me that each of us as souls possess certain genetic coding at the spiritual or soul level. Prior to our incarnation, the soul agrees to and accepts certain attributes, traits, and characteristics as a means of experiencing life and learning from these lessons, which is the ultimate purpose of each incarnation. The DNA blueprint for these genetic attributes has a quantum, multidimensional origin, often referred to as Source. The genetic information represented by these Source codes is embodied in unique quantum light patterns, or frequency arrays, recorded vibrationally on the Akash within our personal quantum field (Merkaba). The Source code is transmitted and informs the DNA information stored in our personal quantum field. It is then interpreted by us in a way that affects our genetic coding. In fact, our genetic response is evidence of the way our consciousness has interpreted this Source code for us. Although there is a default genetic coding that is inherent to each of us, my channels indicate that we can alter the design at will, meaning it is possible to influence our genetic coding if we choose. We can work with consciousness in a way that can alter the frequencies stored in our DNA to change the blueprint information in order to re-encode our genes. The means by which this was accomplished is covered in subsequent chapters.

> **We can work with consciousness in a way that can alter the frequencies stored in our DNA to change the blueprint information in order to re-encode our genes.**

This information also correlates with what Robert Detzler, founder of a very powerful healing technique called Spiritual Restructuring Therapy, describes as potentials that exist in our DNA and chromosomes that are created in the etheric plane prior to incarnation. As stated earlier, the term *potential* means that any number of possible scenarios for expression are possible, depending on a number of factors, including human consciousness. Therefore, at this level, the potential for perfect DNA and chromosomes is represented, but during the process of incarnation, we become less than perfect as our energetic bodies are created. This dysfunction is then carried down and manifested in the physical body. Once the soul decides to incarnate, certain genetic codes are assigned to the DNA blueprint to achieve certain physical results.[1]

He goes on to say that there are many positive qualities that are part of the soul's genetic code, which include attributes such as understanding, love, patience, humility, composure, benevolence, selflessness, clarity, and such. The task of each soul is to acknowledge, appreciate, and learn to use these in a harmonious way so that we can manifest our full spiritual potential. When we fail to do so, we create discordant energy (as thoughts and emotions) that must be cleared in order to promote more positive expression.[2] Discordant energy manifests itself not only in terms of our behaviors and personality, but also at a much deeper physical level in us, including at the cellular and genetic level.

I have been shown in my channeling sessions, through a series of visual metaphors, that we are all cut from the same fabric or genetic origins from Source, but depending on specific light patterns that represent this genetic information, this fabric becomes altered and yields the variation in genetic coding we see at the individual level. The fabric, in my view, is analogous to the Akash, the substance upon which all life is created. The fibers themselves contain the information of this universal whole and the entire spiritual essence (denoted to some as Spirit, the animating force) of everything, in other words, humanity's entire event history as well as the divine plan. This means that all human DNA structure and their potentials are identical. In keeping with the concept of our quantum nature then, we are all aspects of the same thing and are therefore never separate. In fact, when humans are compared with other species "there is a high level of conservation, meaning that all of life shares the same molecular tool kit, with only minor differences being observed, in that the genes are homologous." This is also evidenced by the small number of encoding genes we possess.[3] Therefore, the only thing that differentiates us from each other is the DNA information held holographically as light patterns within our personal quantum field along with that which is held within our own Akashic Records, stored in the quantum portion of our DNA.[4]

TRANSMISSION OF UNIVERSAL GENETIC INFORMATION

My understanding from my channels is that through quantum electromagnetic mechanisms, genetic information originating from Source is conveyed to our personal quantum fields and the DNA information contained there through a "universal communications network,"[5] which exists as part of this nonphysical, multidimensional space. Source genetic codes are transmitted throughout this network via wormholes, which were shown to me as shafts or corridors of light that function as portals connecting with other dimensions. These wormholes transit the space-time continuum, functioning as portals or connections from quantum, multidimensional fields within the universe, including the Akashic Field, into our three-dimensional space. Source genetic code information is transferred from these origins as complex arrays of quantum emissions (photons) or frequencies, which make up holographic light patterns or light codes described earlier. The sun's magnetic field helps to organize and hold these photons in place, through the forces of attraction. The photons inside these wormholes exhibit an inherent or natural resonant frequency, known as a *harmonic oscillation*. This oscillating motion produces pressure that propagates them through the wormhole in wave form. Photons moving in a wave form constitutes an electrical current or signal. A flowing electrical current produces an expanding magnetic field with lines of force at a 90-degree angle to the direction of current flow. When a current increases or decreases, the magnetic field exhibits a corresponding change in the same way. Here, oscillating electrical fields produce magnetic fields, which in turn oscillate to produce another corresponding electrical field. The net effect is the creation of an electromagnetic wave, which, in other words, is light. The waves also create sound due to the variations in pressure change. Thus, quantum genetic information encoded in light and sound waves is transmitted to our personal quantum field and the DNA information contained there.

> **Thus, quantum genetic information encoded in light and sound waves is transmitted to our personal quantum field and the DNA information contained there.**

As it was described to me, a quantum vacuum state exists inside these wormholes, which is also consistent with the explanation of quantum fields and the Zero Point Field provided earlier. Again, the field is not empty, but contains a cosmic medium, the Akash, that transports light, energy, and pressure. Scientific experiments have proven that this quantum vacuum is a physically real medium that interacts with matter and produces real effects. Under vacuum conditions, light does not bend and maintains its integrity, so the integrity of the light information would be preserved. Therefore, the quantum vacuum is really the "holographic information mechanism that records the historical experience of matter" emanating from Source and storing quantum genetic code holographically at a nonlocal level upon the Akash.[6]

The information carried in the vacuum is not localized, confined to a single, specific location only. As in a hologram, the vacuum carries information in distributed form, present at all points where the wave fields [which are wave patterns created by moving waves that intersect and interfere as they travel in a medium] have propagated. The interfering wave fields in the vacuum are natural holograms. They propagate quasi-instantly, and nothing can cancel them. Thus, nature's holograms are cosmic holograms—they link—"in-form"—all things with all other things.[7]

This mechanism of transmission has been demonstrated experimentally by Russian scientists working with DNA in a laboratory. They discovered that it can cause disturbance patterns in a vacuum, producing magnetized wormholes. Wormholes are defined as the microscopic equivalents of the Einstein-Rosen bridges that are found in the vicinity of black holes. Similar to the information received in my channels, they are portrayed as tunnel connections between entirely different areas in the universe through which information can be transmitted outside of space and time. Russian researcher Vladimir Poponin placed DNA in a tube and beamed a laser through it. When the DNA was removed, the laser light continued spiraling on its own, as it would through a crystal. These phantom energy patterns continued to emanate those of the removed DNA, thus exhibiting the "Phantom DNA Effect." Therefore, energy from outside space and time still flows through the activated wormholes even after the DNA is removed.[8] This confirms that the integrity of the Source genetic code as quantum holographic light patterns is preserved and can be transmitted to the DNA contained in our personal quantum field.

As previously indicated, quantum holographic light patterns representing the Source genetic code originating from the universal Akashic Field are transmitted via the wormholes as electrical impulses (quantum emissions) and are charged by the sun's energy and higher frequency cosmic rays. Bundles of filaments, comprised of underlying energy fields, shown to me as being much like fiber-optic cables, emanate from the wormholes, propagating these electrical impulses toward three-dimensional space by sound waves. The filaments turn off and on (by processes known as radiation and occlusion) in accordance with these electrical impulses, creating appropriate sequencing of frequencies that make up a light pattern. These were described as being similar to circuit boards, which are our soul's light patterns (genetic information) that are contained within our personal quantum field. These "circuit boards" make up the information for the DNA blueprint for our body and the map for our genetic attributes, traits, and characteristics.

When the quantum light information pulsed through the wormholes hits the Earth, it is anchored by another magnetic field, created by the Earth's magnetic grid. When the Earth's magnetic field in turn overlaps with the magnetic field generated by us, the transfer of Source genetic code information from the Akashic Field (Source) to our DNA is facilitated. This transfer of information occurs magnetically through inductance when they are entangled enough to communicate. Our genetic coding comes from the activation of these patterns within our personal quantum field based on our quantum DNA's ability to receive and translate the information into instructions for biological functioning tasks within this magnetically coupled environment. This is how quantum genetic information patterns a portion of our DNA that is imprinted on the physical gene structure. The mechanism by which this occurs will be covered in more detail in the following chapter.

> **"**
> When the quantum light information pulsed through the wormholes hits the Earth, it is anchored by another magnetic field, created by the Earth's magnetic grid. When the Earth's magnetic field in turn overlaps with the magnetic field generated by us, the transfer of Source genetic code information from the Akashic Field (Source) to our DNA is facilitated. **"**

Science has shown that weak electromagnetic fields (electric and photonic) have the ability to transmit high amounts of information, or what is referred to as bio-information. Electric fields can affect biological organisms by transmitting electrical information through fluctuation in specific frequencies and amplitudes. What is interesting is that because the weak electromagnetic fields are nonlinear, fields in targeted frequency and amplitude ranges can have large effects.[9] Effectively then, we exist in an electromagnetic field, and such that an alternating current operates within our DNA blinking on and off at the rate of the speed of light. The electrical current flows in one direction to display light, which holds quantum genetic information, and then reverses and flows in the opposite direction, generating a magnetic field, which attracts quantum genetic information.

Experiments showing how electromagnetic frequencies can re-encode DNA molecules in bacteria illustrate this point. In an experiment conducted by Nobel Prize–winner Luc Montagnier, a specific electromagnetic signal emitted by a pathogenic bacterial culture was shown to remain even after the biological material was removed from the culture medium. Even when a new, nonpathogenic strain of the same bacteria was placed in the culture medium having that particular electromagnetic frequency, the new material was transformed into the pathogenic strain, essentially by influencing the DNA molecules of the bacteria and re-coding it.[10]

I have been told through my channels that the influence of this magnetic environment holds the key to unlocking some of the information that encodes our genes and is very important. Researchers have shown that magnetic fields, particularly those existing at extremely low frequencies, have a pronounced effect on virtually all cellular and chemical processes in living things. Some say that cells are, in actual fact, magnetic. This effect is believed to be due to the orientation of molecules and their spin as well as distortion of the angle of molecules in the magnetic field.[11] They have also concluded, through experimentation, that the information transmitted and received by human beings has a strong magnetic component to it.[12] Tests have shown that protein molecules are susceptible to electric and magnetic field modulations and that enzymes also behave differently when subjected to a magnetic field. Cellular and genetic response mechanisms within the context of energetic environments will be described in later chapters.

ANOMALIES IN GENETIC INFORMATION

Our bodies function very much like semiconductors by transmitting electrical flow throughout. We know that a flowing electric current produces expanding magnetic fields at right angles to the direction of the current flow. Minerals in the human body, in their most elemental state as atoms, carry an electrical charge when they are present in this electromagnetic field. There is a weak electric field around each of us, which, according to my channels, is said to exist only when we are connected electrically and likely entangled in a quantum sense to this higher source of frequencies. As long as the electrical circuit remains connected, the Source genetic code in the light patterns is perpetuated in our personal quantum field. If the electrical circuit is interrupted and the signal is parsed, the light patterns are altered and the integrity of the genetic information is disrupted. When our conscious thoughts and emotions create discordant or negative energy in our personal quantum field, they distort these light patterns and influence the information signaled to and interpreted by our DNA. When our personal quantum field energy is affected in this way, we lose access to our original Source genetic coding patterns as they were intended for us. Scientific experiments have verified that when human DNA is isolated and then exposed to the influence of individuals displaying various emotions, the DNA responds by changing its configuration and tensile characteristics.[13] The idea that patterns caused by negative thoughts and emotions, or driven by undesirable subconscious mind or soul programs, may eventually lead to a deleterious cellular and genetic response because of the misinformation that is now being signaled to our DNA will be expounded upon in later chapters.

> When our conscious thoughts and emotions create discordant or negative energy in our personal quantum field, they distort these light patterns and influence the information signaled to and interpreted by our DNA. When our personal quantum field energy is affected in this way, we lose access to our original Source genetic coding patterns as they were intended for us.

This is why clearing the emotional, mental, and spiritual energetic bodies is so critical to our health. As part of my healing process, my practitioners focused heavily on clearing my energy bodies, reducing influence from outside electrical interferences and ensuring that this electrical connectivity was maintained through various means. The work of Dr. Merrill Garnett, prominent cancer researcher, has confirmed the necessity of this alternating electrical current (AC current) in achieving the high efficiency electron transfers needed for biological systems to operate along with life force. "As long as you pulse, energy can traverse great distances with low resistance," he says.[14] This has a profound influence on the electrical properties at a cellular level and, hence, gene response. As we know, there are a myriad of techniques involving energy work and body therapies that all work in various ways to remove the impediments and blocks to energy flow in our bodies and strengthen our electrical flow and, thus, our electromagnetic fields.

Living biological systems are said to be characterized by a kind of complex spectrum of frequencies, where frequencies work and communicate together in a coordinated fashion. Optimal systems are polychromatic, where all frequencies in the spectral range are represented and participating. However, in a nonoptimal or unhealthy state, some of those frequencies may be missing, over-represented, or there may be gaps in the spectrum. Aromatherapy, homeopathy, sound healing, and other forms of vibrational healing modalities work by presenting a specific array of frequencies with a unique energetic signature that the patient may be missing, in order to complete the spectrum or pattern.[15] Healthy biological organisms would therefore exhibit coherent patterns or fields, and conversely, unhealthy ones would be characterized by disruptions or unintegrated signals. According to geneticist Mae-Wan Ho, "when an area of the body stops properly communicating, it will fall back on its own mode of frequency productions, which leads to an impoverishment of its frequency spectrum."[16] When there are frequency anomalies or irregularities in these arrays of light, they create a less-than-perfect result that ultimately translates as alterations in genetic coding, as will be explained in further detail in subsequent chapters.

Therefore, maintaining a strong electrical flow in the body is critical to ensuring we are an appropriate host so that the transmission of genetic information can take place as was intended from Source, without distortions or anomalies.

DNA AS RECEIVERS

My channels also indicate that our physical DNA, and the strands themselves, act as vibrational receptors or antenna for sound. This function as an electromagnetic receiver and transmitter is actually more important in affecting cellular and genetic response than the protein synthesis function that is traditionally described by science. Some scientists believe that "chromosomes work like holographic bio-computers, using the DNA's own electromagnetic radiation to generate and interpret spiraling waves of sound and light that run up and down the DNA ladder."[17] The DNA's unique helical structure is like an antenna in which the long linear polymer structure is suited for receiving and transmitting electrical impulses, while the ring formed from the cross-section of the spiraling double helix is appropriate for magnetic impulses.[18] The combination of the electrical and magnetic forces creates an electromagnetic field. It appears that not only can DNA receive, transduce, and interpret signals, it can elicit a response and re-emit electromagnetic signals. It is thought that DNA may also be able to do so with Zero Point Field energy and interact more directly with quantum fields in this way.[19] This has been confirmed by the wave-based genome theory devised by Russian scientists, which suggests that the physical DNA functions simultaneously as a source and receiver of language "texts" constructed in a specific way. They also believe that the chromosome itself acts like a holographic grating that dynamically displays or transduces light and electroacoustic fields.[20]

Quantum information is broadcast through the universe carried by sound waves, upon which universal or quantum genetic information is stored holographically. There is an entire spectrum of frequencies, which we can think of like radio stations, each with their own unique frequency. Our DNA functions like radio receiver antennas, tuning in to the various stations, picking up the sound waves. When the DNA is "attuned" to a particular station—in other words, when DNA and the station resonate at the same frequency—the wave information is decoded by our DNA in a very specific way. Thus, DNA "is the 'antenna' of body orchestration and takes that which is multidimensional and converts it into information, then action."[21]

It has also been suggested that because DNA is a quantum harmonic oscillator, it produces particles known as *phonons*. Long wavelength phonons produce sound, so the DNA strand, which is believed to be light encoded, is actually an electrotonal filament. Similar to the mechanism by which the Source genetic code is transferred as light and sound through magnetically coupled fields described earlier, physical DNA may also be facilitating quantum communication in the same manner.[22] According to some, presumably these filaments, activated by waves of energized sound and light can literally switch genes on and off.[23] We will return to expound on this concept in more detail in later chapters.

DNA responds to both inaudible and audible sounds and, of particular note, to the sound of one's own voice. This was proven scientifically, where language frequencies such as words (which are sounds) were used successfully to repair damaged DNA.[24] Coincidentally, the basic structure of the alkaline base pairs of our DNA follows regular grammar and set rules about the way words are put together (syntax) and their meaning (semantics), similar to human languages.[25] Therefore, DNA is not only responsible for the development and function of our bodies, but also serves as data storage and communication. "One revolutionary implication of Gariaev's research [speaking of Russian biophysicist and molecular biologist Pyotr Gariaev] is that you can simply use words and sentences of any human language to modulate DNA" frequency emissions. During one experiment, live DNA, that is DNA in living tissue, responded to "language-modulated laser beams and even radio waves. This response was frequency dependent and frequency specific. In this way, the investigators theoretically explained how and why healing affirmations and hypnotherapies have such strong effects."[26] We will examine the effects of sound healing on DNA further in a later chapter.

Many of my channels have also suggested that water plays a role in the transmission and storage of genetic information, which is corroborated by the theory that "genetic inheritance is energetically transmitted bio-acoustically and electromagnetically through special water molecules that form the electromagnetic matrix of DNA."[27] Water conducts sound four times faster than air, and because our bodies are made up of 70 percent water, it is likely that it plays some role in entraining the sound waves.

As we know, sound moves in waves and in turn creates fields. Particular sounds are passed into, out of, and through the body through molecules, which act as transfer points for information. A molecule can literally take on the vibration of an initial pulse and pass this vibration on to its neighbors, which is why sound can shape and change the body and its fields. Water molecules, formed from crystals, will actually shape and reshape according to the vibration of a sound or the information coded into it.[28]

Scientists have demonstrated that water molecules create what is referred to as *coherent domains,* which exhibit a high degree of order and organization. Photons in water have a high degree of coherence, which allows them to exhibit single wavelength characteristics. These appear to become "informed" in the presence of other molecules by polarizing around any charged molecule, storing and carrying its frequency so that it may be read at a distance. In other words, patterns are encoded in the water. "This would mean that water has memory and is like a tape recorder, imprinting and carrying energetic information whether the original molecule is still there or not."[29] Therefore, water may be essential in the transmission and storage of energy patterns and information in the body. Interestingly, studies have revealed that dolphins and whales are capable of transmitting sound signals and generating electromagnetic fields that can affect human DNA.[30] Through our DNA, "our cells are engaged with every other body part through light and sound-based resonant signaling."[31]

Certain frequencies generated by acoustic or electromagnetic fields can change the structure of water. When water becomes structured, its surface tension is lowered, which my channels indicate is the mechanism by which physical DNA is actually modified. Chromosomes are in fact surrounded by a layer of water, and as the structure of the water changes, the shape of the DNA can change. The work of Igor Smirnov has demonstrated that membrane layers surrounding the nucleus of the cell make it difficult to introduce agents that could modify gene expression. According to Smirnov, structured water, in contrast, can easily reach the nucleus and can carry information and change the genetic code and influence different patterns of gene expression depending on their energy status.[32]

QUANTUM DNA
AS STORAGE DEVICES

According to my channels, Source genetic codes in the form of quantum holographic light patterns are stored in the crystalline structure of our physical DNA. Crystals, as we know, store energetic information and retain energy pattern memory as vibration. Scientists have indicated that the reason DNA can store light is because it is an aperiodic crystal, exhibiting patterns that are not periodic or regular, but rather those that are quasi-periodic, which can be indicative of its quantum character. Recent research has shown it is possible for a quantum memory, which means something that can store and recall information, to be able to store photonic information in a crystal with reasonable efficiency.[33]

The actual sheath that is wrapped around the DNA molecule is crystalline in nature and contains the memory of our entire event history, including our Akashic Record. Our DNA blueprint is also held within this memory. In other words, the coding for our entire life—everything we have been, are, or will become on all levels—is held within the crystalline structure of our DNA.[34]

> **In other words, the coding for our entire life—everything we have been, are, or will become on all levels—is held within the crystalline structure of our DNA.**

The experiment by Russian scientists Pyotr Gariaev and Vladimir Poponin, referred to previously, proved that DNA is capable of forming and holding structure in energy. When they placed photons in a vacuum tube with DNA, the random photons became orderly (coherent), taking on the structure of the DNA. When they removed the DNA from the vacuum tube, the photons remained orderly for more than a month.[35] A physicist by the name of Fritz-Albert Popp also demonstrated that tiny frequencies are stored and emitted from the DNA of cells. Interestingly, the emission intensity of the light remained stable until the organism was disturbed or ill, at which point the current went sharply up or down. Cancer victims that were studied actually had fewer photons.[36]

> **Thus, the instructions for our genetic coding are contained within the two strands of our physical DNA, while the memory of who we are in terms of our Akashic Record and DNA blueprint is contained in the crystalline structure of the other ten strands of quantum, multidimensional DNA, held as a band of frequencies.**

Thus, the instructions for our genetic coding are contained within the two strands of our physical DNA, while the memory of who we are in terms of our Akashic Record and DNA blueprint is contained in the crystalline structure of the other ten strands of quantum, multidimensional DNA, held as a band of frequencies. Our physical DNA and our quantum DNA are in constant communication and inform each other in a way that translates the genetic code to generate a cellular and genetic response. A measure of the efficiency with which this communication takes place is referred to as our *DNA efficiency*, a concept that we will return to in a later chapter.

QUANTUM AND BIOLOGICAL
INHERITANCE COMBINED

None of us are born into this world as souls with a completely blank slate. We do not start over each time we incarnate, and the knowledge and experience we have acquired is cumulative. As previously stated, each individual soul has a personal Akashic Record that is stored holographically as memory in the crystalline structure of their DNA. The Akashic Records are much like a repository or library of knowledge, accessed through our consciousness, which holds the key to the true essence of who we are as souls—past, present, and future. This record contains the event history of everything a soul has experienced—all thoughts, emotions, expressions, and actions, from the beginning of creation, throughout our past lives up to the present moment and beyond. It is not a record of our past lives in the linear way that we might imagine it. Instead, it exists as memory and is a nonlocal record imprinted energetically in our physical DNA.

> This record within the DNA contains the interdimensional aspects of personal energy delivery, for it helps to posture who you are in each lifetime, apart from the biological, 3D chemistry contained in the protein-encoded portions of the DNA. This record is contained in the quantum, random chemistry and is not a linear representation of past lives. Instead, it is an "instruction set to connect to the main library," which is in a quantum state in what you would perceive as another dimension . . . there is an idea that the Human's Akashic Record is somehow physically contained in the DNA. It isn't; only "pointers to the library" are there. But even pointers take up 3D space within the Human Genome.[37]

Therefore, there is a component of Akashic Inheritance that stems from our soul's records, which is the quantum complement to our biological inheritance. It is nonlocal information, representing the nonencoded portion of DNA, containing our spiritual blue-print and an imprint of the information for who we are. Although we acquire biologically inherited DNA traits from the chemistry of our parents, the largest traits of our personality are carried in the Akashic Records.[38]

Although we acquire biologically inherited DNA traits from the chemistry of our parents, the largest traits of our personality are carried in the Akashic Records.

Robert Detzler says that "you do not inherit disease, you inherit beliefs. These are the beliefs of a person's parents and grandparents as far back as nine generations. They are in the genes." He says that inheritance is actually "a spiritual version of the holographic principle where every part contains the whole," consistent with what has been described earlier. Each of our cells, therefore, contains the whole soul record and programs of a particular person, including their beliefs, which are passed on through the sperm and egg of the parents to become part of the cellular memory of their offspring. Thus, if we inherited a belief about a particular disease from one of our parents and experience situations and events that reinforce these beliefs, we may very well express these by manifesting this as disease. It is possible to clear this genetic programming from cellular memory so that we are free of these inherited messages, as long as we do not consciously rebuild them by listening to other people's beliefs.[39]

Each of us personally has one or two lessons that are assigned to us to accomplish in our lifetime, which we have agreed to by choice and with our soul's permission prior to incarnation. These are unique to us and can vary considerably—they may be about love, compassion, facing the challenges of adversity or a lack of abundance, for instance. Through the mechanism described, these are imprinted as a light pattern on the crystalline portion of our DNA. These patterns become the energetic framework in which we interpret information through our consciousness as we move throughout our lives.

Some of us, like myself, agreed to experience a particular disease as part of our learning process. Sometimes, they can be part of our soul's plan to experience a wide range of circumstances from which to grow and evolve. This is true, even with diseases or conditions that are severely debilitating or even terminal. For example, if the soul needs to face the challenge of a Down's Syndrome-affected body or the stigma of alopecia (a condition for baldness) or some other form of limited body, they would encode these factors into the genetic information that would cause the parents to produce such a body for the soul's needed and chosen experience.[40]

The energy of these programs is stored in our Akashic Records and in our DNA. They can be reinforced by our belief about genetics and that these types of diseases are inherited, cementing their presence in our reality. I was quite astounded when I learned that we are indeed co-creators of our own reality in this way, by choosing what we want to experience. It is important, in putting our lives in perspective then, to understand that we are not victims of our lives but, to a large degree, designers of it.[41] However, because of the fact that we were in part responsible for choosing these lessons, as we evolve and grow as a soul, we need to be reminded that we also have the capacity to change these agreements, thereby changing the information our consciousness interprets and, thus, what we express genetically.

> **❝**
> It is important, in putting our lives in perspective then, to understand that we are not victims of our lives but, to a large degree, designers of it. However, because of the fact that we were in part responsible for choosing these lessons, as we evolve and grow as a soul, we need to be reminded that we also have the capacity to change these agreements, thereby changing the information our consciousness interprets and, thus, what we express genetically. **❞**

According to Kryon, the angelic energy channeled through Lee Carroll, we also have "galactic Akashic Inheritance." There are races from other planets, dimensions, and universes including the Pleidians, Andromedans, and Arcturians who have seeded our quantum or spiritual DNA with the wisdom of the past and our true spiritual nature. They have been described as our ancestors and spiritual parents and grandparents.[42] Many who channel entities from these origins, confirm their interest and support in assisting humans in our spiritual awakening and survival. They are here to remind us of what so many of us have forgotten as we are caught up in our daily quest for healing, meaning, and purpose in our lives. We are not separate from Oneness; we have simply forgotten so that we may learn our soul's lessons. We hold the expression of the divine and this universal Akashic intelligence in every cell. This is also inscribed in our DNA.

Therefore, in addition to our biological inheritance, we also inherit quantum traits based on our spiritual origins and what is held in our Akashic Records as well as our divine plan. These have an unbelievably powerful influence in defining who we are and what we manifest in our lives, including disease. Our DNA is based on a combination of both our biological (chemical) and quantum (spiritual) inheritance. Together, these define our energetic as well as our physical bodies. The biological portion of our DNA contains the genomic instructions, while the quantum portion contains the drivers that make those instructions work. Both work together to influence genetic coding. When we understand what is held in our DNA in terms of both of these, we can easily see how profoundly it governs the deepest aspects of our lives, our beliefs, behaviors, actions, and choices as well as our health by the information that is communicated.

Not only can we access the Akashic Field to obtain wisdom, knowledge, and guidance, we can also work with the vibrational energies that reside there to expand our consciousness and heal. We can access the energy of our soul's entire event history and work with it to achieve our highest good in health, wellness, and in manifesting our true potential in our present lives. In this manner, we activate DNA that was previously hidden and dormant and can bring about complete changes in our genetic coding and our health. These energies may be invisible and unmeasurable at this time, but they contain the most amazing opportunities we have to heal, by changing the information contained within our DNA and thus by re-encoding our genes, which most have previously considered unalterable.

Some souls are designed to complete this assignment within a lifetime and will regain their health, others are simply acquiring an experience on the overall continuum of self-mastery. In other words, for certain individuals, if disease is their soul's chosen path in this particular incarnation, they may not necessarily respond to any form of physical intervention, healing energies, or attempts to adjust their DNA, for a designated period of time or throughout their entire lifetime. Their illness condition is seen as an undertaking that most often serves either the individual or the greater community or society in some way, as an experience. Even if disease is a result (in whole or in part) of specific energetic blocks associated with core ancestral wounds or soul programs, full recovery may not always be achieved within an individual's lifetime. Success in this regard depends largely on their willingness and ability to work through, release, and transform these energies. However, as we will see for most, through various consciousness tools, if we so choose, it is entirely possible to create whatever changes are necessary to improve health outcomes and even revert the body back to its original nondisease state by re-encoding our genes.

> **Not only can we access the Akashic Field to obtain wisdom, knowledge, and guidance, we can also work with the vibrational energies that reside there to expand our consciousness and heal. We can access the energy of our soul's entire event history and work with it to achieve our highest good in health, wellness, and in manifesting our true potential in our present lives.**

4

DNA Interaction
with Quantum Information
The Quantum Interface

The field is there. Contact with it releases power.

LAUREL ELIZABETH KEYES[1]

MECHANISM OF QUANTUM
INFORMATION TRANSFER

As previously indicated in my channels, the key to understanding the interaction between us and our quantum environment is through magnetics. In fact, the mechanism by which nonlocal quantum genetic information is transferred to our DNA and our cells is through the process of inductance, which is a form of magnetic coupling. This represents a slight departure from the most currently accepted scientific theory that maintains information transfer occurs through resonance and, more specifically, through a process called *phase adaptive conjugate resonance* (PCAR). To reiterate, from the quantum vacuum theory, we know that a wave field, which is a field created from oscillating waves of quantum emissions, that encounters another wave field will create an interference pattern, which is the quantum hologram. When these two wave fields are coupled with each other (conjugate), they begin to vibrate at the same frequency, which is the condition known as resonance. PCAR is described as a kind of selective resonance in which the individualized wave fields create a spatially and temporally coherent channel of communication between them that can transfer nonlocal information.[2]

Rather, when the personal quantum field that surrounds around us and our DNA overlaps with a nonlocal, universal Akashic Field of information, they become attuned to each other when the band of frequencies contained within the crystalline structure of our DNA resonates at the same frequency as those of the nonlocal universal Akashic Field. When these two quantum fields overlap, electrical current flowing through our personal quantum field is transmitted through the magnetic field that develops as a result of the current flow, creating a condition known as *inductance*. Inductance involves the expansion or contraction of the magnetic field. As the magnetic field varies, it causes an electromotive force that provides a stabilizing effect by opposing any further change in the electrical current flowing through it. In other words, inductance is the process by which the flow of electrical charge is impeded by the temporary storage of energy as a magnetic field. Inductance can occur without two objects physically touching each other (such as two quantum fields in proximity to each other). Inductance also amplifies the electrical potential of the energy. Electrical impulses or arcs, created by the spin of quantum particles (photons) as described, pass between the fields when they are in high magnetic resonance with each other. When these two fields are mutually inductively coupled (magnetically coupled), the Source genetic code information as quantum holographic light patterns are transferred from one field to the other when conductance reaches its maximum. This mechanism is consistent with the theory of inductive coupling described by science.

> When these two quantum fields overlap, electrical current flowing through our personal quantum field is transmitted through the magnetic field that develops as a result of the current flow, creating a condition known as *inductance*.

According to the information provided in my channels, this mechanism does not occur by happenstance, but rather a form of what was described to me as organized entropy, which is sometimes referred to as "hidden energy." With organized entropy, a form of overall order or coherence arises naturally from the interactions between parts of a system showing disorder—in this case, when the two separate quantum fields exhibiting entropy (fluctuating electrical current) overlap. The interaction of the two fields, when inductively coupled, results in the self-organization of the information contained within the fields spontaneously, which is amplified by any positive feedback. This creates a condition of decentralization, which is more robust and enduring, in other words, more coherent. Therefore, the mechanism yields a trend toward order, or coherence, as opposed to disorder. Higher vibrational states therefore yield greater electrical impulses and coherence in quantum emissions or holographic light information and, thus, represent a more effective means of information transfer and communication. "Coherence establishes communication. It's like a subatomic telephone network. The better the coherence, the finer the telephone network and the more refined wave patterns [that] have a telephone."[3] Scientist Herbert Frolich demonstrated that "once energy reaches a certain threshold, molecules begin to vibrate in unison until they reach a high level of coherence. The moment molecules reach this state of coherence, they take on certain qualities of quantum mechanics, including nonlocality. They get to a point where they can operate in tandem."[4]

The process of communication has been described as being between "DNA loops" within this quantum environment, which has a magnetic component to it. Apparently, "each loop of DNA has a magnetic field that overlaps the loop next to it, which overlaps the loop next to it. Trillions of overlaps equals one [single] consciousness. This then represents a magnetic imprint, which Humans [carry] around with them."[5]

Since our physical DNA is shaped like helical coils, they most likely function as inductor coils and exhibit superconducting properties.[6] The shape creates a magnetic field as the current flow expands across adjacent coil turns. If the current changes, the induced magnetic field changes, creating a force called the *counter EMF*, which stabilizes additional changes in current. This is the exact same inductance phenomenon described earlier. This counter EMF effect only occurs during dynamic current fluctuations characteristic of alternating electrical current (AC) circuits and not when the current is static, as in direct current (DC) circuits. As previously stated, physical DNA has a crystalline structure that is conducive to transferring electrical impulses and, thus, Source genetic code information as quantum holographic light patterns. This explains why the DNA contained in our cells allows them to receive the same message about purpose and function (genetic information) without being physically adjacent to each other. When we view DNA in the context of its energetic environment, it can be seen as an intercellular communication system. As scientist Steve Haltiwanger points out, "normal multicellular organisms require coherent and coordinated communication with the other cells in the organism. In order to synchronize cellular process in a multicellular state, a communication system must exist."[7]

Bruce Lipton, author of *The Biology of Belief*, writes:

Hundreds upon hundreds of scientific studies of the last fifty years have consistently revealed that "invisible forces" of the electromagnetic spectrum profoundly impact every facet of biological regulation. These energies include microwaves, radio frequencies, the visible light spectrum, extremely low frequencies, acoustic frequencies, and even a newly recognized form of force known as scalar energy. Specific frequencies and patterns of electromagnetic radiation regulate DNA, RNA, and protein synthesis, alter protein shape and function; and control gene regulation, cell division, cell differentiation, morphogenesis . . . hormone secretion and nerve growth and function.[8]

Because DNA is also quantum and capable of transmitting energetic information to our cells, our physical DNA strands function as our cellular antennas into multidimensional fields, capable of extracting and pulling this information to us for interpretation and use. "The level of consciousness of your cells is determined by their cellular vibration. The higher your cellular vibration, the more strands of DNA, your cellular antenna you activate. . . . So the smallest unit of your physical, your cells, can access the collective or super-consciousness of the universe. More vibration accesses more universal information."[9]

DNA COMMUNICATION THROUGH OUR CONSCIOUSNESS

As Kryon, channeled through Lee Carroll, points out, the key to creating change in the human body is through information, not by altering our chemistry.[10] The expanded view of DNA presented here clearly takes us beyond the idea that our biological DNA consists only of physical protein complexes existing somewhere inside of our bodies, containing codes that control the expression of certain genetic traits and physical attributes, as well as our propensity to medical conditions and disease. Instead, it is information about our quantum genetic inheritance that is communicated to us via our consciousness, in addition to our biological inheritance that encodes our genes and makes us who we are.

> **"**
> **It is information about our quantum genetic inheritance that is communicated to us via our consciousness, in addition to our biological inheritance that encodes our genes and makes us who we are. "**

DNA communicates to you and your consciousness in a different way than your brain does. . . . Information carried in your DNA has to get to your brain eventually in order for you to cognize it [become aware and believe it]. It then arrives in your consciousness and works in a certain way. . . . It does so with what we call overlapping multidimensional fields. . . . DNA doesn't talk to you in memory, synapse, structure, or linearity, it talks to you in emotional concepts.[11]

Without delving into a more detailed examination of consciousness, in order to appreciate that this is even possible, we must accept at the very least that the consciousness is not a physical process that involves activity of neural networks within the brain. Our consciousness is not controlled by the brain or the genes. Instead, it is controlled by the subconsciousness of an Akashic experience.[12] In other words, it is driven by the information contained in our Akashic Records, our event history.

We alter our DNA through conscious intent. DNA doesn't just evolve or change on its own, regardless of what influences might be exerted upon it; it waits for us to direct it. This is a very important distinction: other healing modalities, in my observation, typically adopt more passive approaches that do not purposefully direct the body through our DNA to elicit a response. They are not necessarily targeted at activating the spiritual portion of our DNA that holds the key to our DNA blueprint and our biological instructions.

> **We alter our DNA through conscious intent. DNA doesn't just evolve or change on its own, regardless of what influences might be exerted upon it; it waits for us to direct it.**

In the same way as cellular and DNA communication is triggered by quantum events (such as wave propagation, interference, and magnetic field interaction) as we have described, consciousness also seems to function at the quantum level, enabling it to extend its influence, unbound by time and space. This means through our consciousness we have access to information in the past, present, and future through the Akashic Records. We relate to this information through our thoughts and emotions, which are driven by this Akashic energy. Through our consciousness, then, we have access to Source genetic code information that we can draw upon and apply to our personal quantum field. Providing new information changes and enhances the DNA information as well as the efficiency with which this information is communicated to our cells and our biological DNA instruction sets. This, ultimately, allows us to re-encode our genes.

> Through our consciousness, then, we have access to Source genetic code information that we can draw upon and apply to our personal quantum field. Providing new information changes and enhances the DNA information as well as the efficiency with which this information is communicated to our cells and our biological DNA instruction sets. This, ultimately, allows us to re-encode our genes.

THE INNATE SELF

Our DNA interacts with our consciousness through our Innate Self or "smart body" as it is known, which is contained within our personal quantum field. It represents the bridge between our cellular structure, our DNA, and our consciousness and so is an inseparable part of us.[13] Through my channels, I am told that our "innateness" comes from our "knowingness," not of who we are in a general sense, but who we are unto ourselves. Self relates to the divine within and, therefore, only comes from Source. Innateness predisposes one to the truth of our own inherent divinity. They tell me that innateness swipes a layer of "individual-ness" upon our cells, which is unique to each of us, and that, in this way, we direct ourselves only unto ourselves (internally and uniquely). In other words, no one else marches to the beat of the same drum. Innate has its own intelligence that is separate from what is generated by our brain. Only our Innate knows what we and our bodies need to fulfill our soul's divine purpose in this life and for us be healthy. Our Innate is involved in our spiritual survival, the prime directive for the human soul.[14] We have a relationship with our Innate, and it knows everything about us at the quantum, spiritual, and physical level—it knows what is best for us. It knows what we are allergic to or what supplements and medications might be supportive to us and those that might be harmful. "Innate is aware of all things at the cellular level and is broadcasting all the time. It broadcasts so well that it flows into that which you call the Merkaba [personal quantum field]."[15] Our cells seem to react to our sense of innateness because they respond when we recognize when we are "home" and are thus able to bring us back into a state of balance and health. However, if one switch in this governing mechanism malfunctions, as we will see happened in my case, we lose the connectivity to send a clear message of this to our cells.

The majority of people could not reasonably be expected to work with the complex quantum energies that influence our biology and lie outside our own mental capacity and our linear, three-dimensional reality. Fortunately, as it turns out, we actually do not need to know exactly how to do this to achieve health or well-being because our Innate Self does. We are communicating with our Innate when we employ techniques such as muscle testing, osteopathy, bodywork, body talk, Emotional Freedom Technique (EFT) tapping, and positive verbal affirmations.[16] The consciousness tools presented later in this book are also ways that we can work with our Innate to effect positive change in our bodies. All of these techniques access the internal intelligence of the body (Innate) using conscious intent and deliberate action to elicit a favorable and beneficial energetic, emotional, and ultimately, physical response. The responses are indicative of our Innate's capacity to resynchronize the body-being and return body function to a steady and healthy state in response to our communicated desire. As our Akashic memory and DNA become activated during the re-encoding process described throughout the book and more multidimensional energy (information about our event history) is at our disposal, the Innate becomes more proficient in its ability to respond effectively. In other words, as Lee Carroll points out, "the wiser we are, the better we act, and the greater chance of survival we have."[17]

At a deeper level, Innate oversees our biological affairs by controlling all of our cellular instructions and behaving much like a central processing unit for our genes.

> Innate knows everything chemically that's going on in your body. . . . Innate is what sorts out the information in your stem cells. . . . Every piece of DNA in you is absolutely identical and unique. They have your chemical and quantum imprint . . . your DNA, these identical pieces, work together in a way that has not been discovered yet . . . , there is an intelligence that is not what our brain is producing. Your Innate gives information to a very tiny percent of the DNA chemistry, which then makes the genes of the Human body. The stem cells are the templates for these genes. The engine of the race car that propels your body around life is only 3 percent of DNA. 90 percent is the blueprint that is the template for the race engine. Innate is smart and intelligent. It's what we call "body intelligence." . . . Innate can instruct your body to build a better engine, and the blueprints are there for it . . . perfect stem cell blueprints are in your DNA.[18]

Since living cells in any organism evolve and grow from more simple stem cells, the phenomenon of quantum entanglement may explain the mechanism by which information about the whole organism is carried in the quantum attributes of its smaller parts, in accordance with the quantum holographic principle. Cells can become highly specialized and orchestrate extremely complex functioning in the body when all the DNA information is shared by quantum means—ubiquitously and instantaneously.

The fact that the vital body systems can continue to function even after a spinal cord injury, which effectively severs the brain's connection with the body, is evidence of the existence of a system of governance outside the brain. This is the Innate Self's role. Innate is responsible for the seemingly mysterious and miraculous healings—accelerated recoveries, spontaneous remissions, and unexplained disappearances of incurable diseases. There is no mystery after all when the Innate is involved and can bridge the gap between quantum intelligent information that holds all the answers and our bodies.[19] It is not a force outside ourselves—it is something within all of us.

However, as smart and capable as our Innate Self is, it rests in autopilot and plays a default set of instructions to our cells, unless we communicate our desire for something different. One of the most empowering aspects of our ability to self-heal is that we are able to gain permission from our Innate to work with the energies contained in our Akash to activate the quantum portion of our DNA and the memory stored within our DNA's crystalline structure. With the involvement and permission from our Innate as the overseer of our body's and cell's affairs, we can access the DNA information we need to heal, to rid ourselves of disease, and as I discovered, to override any detrimental influence from our biological genes by re-encoding our genes. Our DNA cannot initiate any action of its own accord. It is reactive, not proactive, and changing the messages we provide to it is key.[20]

When our consciousness can communicate with our quantum DNA via the Innate, we can now begin to see the enormous influence we have over the information we provide to our cells, which ultimately influence our genes.

Every time a cell reproduces to make another one, there is a query within the division process. That is to say, a question is asked . . . Innate is the one doing the asking and answering, "Do I make a copy of this one or go to the blueprint?" And the question is answered by this question: "Is there new information?" The answer, "No, make a copy."[21]

In the absence of new information, our DNA will default to the existing programs, messages defined by our existing biological and quantum (spiritual) inheritance. Conveniently, scientific experiments have shown that DNA operates like a language, and so we can communicate with it without decoding. It will respond to us as a result of us simply talking to it. This observation is critical to our understanding and appreciation of the fact that we can influence and reprogram our genes by introducing new information to our DNA in the form of words and frequencies, without having to physically alter our genes.[22] Our Innate is ready to access the information that is appropriate for us and is waiting for our instruction. Through our consciousness then, it is possible to override any erroneous DNA information that may have altered our genetic coding and instruct our DNA to translate the information in our blueprint differently for a more desirable genetic outcome.

> **DNA operates like a language, and so we can communicate with it without decoding. It will respond to us as a result of us simply talking to it.**

What's more, as the world evolves and human consciousness expands, more and more of this DNA is enabled. "Your consciousness, Innate, and your Higher Self are ready to create a body which does not age as much, and where you don't need to worry as much about disease. It's more than just chemistry. It's consciousness over matter."[23]

THE HIGHER SELF

As previously mentioned, our Higher Self is also contained within our personal quantum field and has a role to play in the interaction between consciousness and our DNA. Our Higher Self is the most spiritually evolved aspect of our being and represents the divinity within and our "godlike" self. It is seen as a portal to the most sacred part of who we are and provides us access to nonlocal, multidimensional realms. The Higher Self is the overseer of our lives and can see into our past, present, and future. It works by integrating with our human self and becoming its vehicle of consciousness. Our Higher Self provides inner teaching and guidance to assist us in evolving spiritually, which is achieved when our conscious awareness expands as we learn through the consequences of the choices and actions we exercise in our life experiences. The Higher Self is objective and has our best interests at heart, no matter how we feel about ourselves, whether we think we are capable of healing or not. When we step out of a subjective, self-centered ego state and relinquish our desire to control our lives and our health and surrender ourselves to our Higher Self, we have an opportunity to heal and transform. By consciously invoking our Higher Self to participate in the healing process in concert with our Innate Self, we are deferring to a greater source of knowledge and wisdom that knows exactly what is for our best and highest good and what we need in order to heal and can communicate this directly to our DNA. We are inviting the insight that is most often needed into our awareness that fuels the impetus for change and healing. Through our consciousness, we are able to bring the more ethereal, intangible aspects of our divinity into a more tangible and active relationship with our human self to manifest the changes we desire.

5

Energy of the Subconscious Mind and Soul That Shapes Our DNA

We Are Soul and Self-Made

All illness has its origin in a disharmony between the mind and the spirit levels of the entity and that of the universal pattern for the entity. Thus healing at the physical or even the etheric level is only temporary if the basic pattern at the mind and spirit level remains unchanged.

WILLIAM TILLER[1]

THE SUBCONSCIOUS MIND AND SOUL

From a more spiritual perspective, according to Robert Detzler, we actually have twelve nonphysical, energetic bodies in addition to our physical body. They include the more commonly known ones such as the etheric, astral, mental, emotional, and soul bodies, among others. These bodies have numerous subconscious and conscious minds— the conscious mind functions as the working consciousness of a body and the subconscious mind as the recording device for the experience of the body. He says that the physical body is a lower vibratory expression of our greater self, and the subconscious mind of our physical body records all the beliefs, perceptions, judgments, and experiences of our conscious minds. The origins of these beliefs can be cultural; religious or faith based; situational; or those we acquire through the experience of daily life. We embody these in our attitudes, actions, and behaviors. When the body dies, the conscious and subconscious minds also die, and the vibrational records that were previously held in the subconscious mind are moved to our soul's Akashic Record.[2] Thus, we inscribe the energy of these beliefs vibrationally on the Akash, within our Akashic Record, which is stored as memory within the crystalline portion of our DNA.

The subconscious mind has an immensely powerful influence over us and shapes our lives in many ways. It gathers information through our senses on various experiences in our external world and bodies, based on the makeup of our soul, its purpose and programs, then forms ideas, perceptions, and judgments and stores them. All of this is done without the involvement or awareness of the conscious mind.

In reality, the subconscious mind is an emotionless database of stored programs, whose function is strictly concerned with reading environmental signals and engaging in hardwired behavioral programs, with no questions asked or judgments made. The subconscious mind is similar to a programmable "hard drive" into which our life experiences are downloaded. The programs are functionally equivalent to hardwired stimulus-response behaviors. Behavior activating stimuli may be signals the nervous system detects from the external world and/or signals that arise from within the body such as emotions, pleasure, and pain. When a stimulus is perceived, it will automatically engage the behavioral response that was learned when the signal was first experienced.[3]

The subconscious mind is strictly a stimulus-response playback device; there is no "ghost" in that part of the "machine" to ponder the long-term consequences of the programs we engage. The subconscious works only in the "now." Consequently, programmed misperceptions in our subconscious mind are not "monitored" and will habitually engage us in inappropriate and limiting behavior.[4]

At a more subliminal level, according to Detzler, we are influenced by what are termed "soul programs" that were originally registered in the subconscious mind, sometimes during traumatic events or during emotionally charged times. The energy of these events is subsequently recorded in our soul's Akashic Records. These programs cover a whole host of issues including beliefs about inheritance, which may come from our parent's genes; believing and accepting other's beliefs; beliefs about who we think we are; a message or belief we received during a stressful occurrence; phobias or deep-seated beliefs acquired as a result of an experience or trauma; beliefs about our worthiness or imperfection (particularly in our body); self-punishing ideas and the like.[5]

Soul programs can exist that have negative energies associated with emotions of anger, hate, or revenge, generated as the result of something a soul has experienced while out of the physical body, particularly during a traumatic event such as rape or another situation involving the infliction of bodily violence. The energy of these experiences is likewise recorded directly into the soul's Akashic Records and not in the conscious or subconscious mind. Other programs include beliefs that tend to separate or polarize (good and evil; God and the devil); astrological beliefs creating destructive behaviors (such as fear); loss of subconscious integrity (by discordant thoughts, emotions, or beliefs that compromise the subconscious mind); scarring (as a result of the soul being wounded and healed); old wives' tales (unfounded information that controls behaviors); and a desire to escape (responsibility, pain, challenge, or difficulty).[6]

There are also soul programs formed during our beginnings in the spiritual realms and before we moved into the physical world as part of the incarnation process that contain energies stored in our Akashic Records. This programming, which contains both positive and negative aspects, is an integral part of each soul's makeup and spiritual body that assists us in relearning what we have forgotten as we make our way along our life's journey, back toward ultimate spiritual consciousness and reconnection with Oneness. A multitude of these programs, some of them quite esoteric, make up the basic architecture of the soul. These are in place as challenges for us, otherwise there would be no opportunity for the soul to perfect itself as it follows its incarnational path. Programs that create dysfunctional thoughts and expressions as discordant energy are opportunities for us to learn, grow, and then ideally move on from these experiences.[7]

Other anomalies that are also registered as part of the soul's energy include energies associated with soul fragmentation and soul loss. Trauma, oaths, vows, and soul contracts between souls, as a few examples, can all influence the memories and perspective that a soul carries forward as energy and can have a major impact on who we are and what we manifest. During my own personal healing journey and work with practitioners during a number of treatment sessions, I experienced the retrieval of my own soul, the return of several of my soul pieces held by others, as well as the release of soul parts I was holding that belonged to others under such arrangements. As a practitioner working in this area, I have witnessed firsthand the profound role that soul energy has on influencing our subconscious beliefs and the energy in our personal quantum field. Matters of the soul are often the root of many dysfunctional patterns we exhibit, both behaviorally and physically. They detract from the ability to achieve completeness as an individual and our true potential and can ultimately lead to the demise of our health and result in disease. It is impossible to dismiss their importance when I have personally felt and witnessed such pronounced and noticeable shifts in others during circumstances when the soul is reconstituted and returns back to its intended state of wholeness. Appreciable changes in people's personalities, relationships, choices, and attitudes, as well as their health occur.

The problem is that the subconscious mind and soul are nondiscriminating and do not monitor what is happening to us on the conscious level when we are not consciously aware or spiritually awakened. Because we are so heavily influenced by these programs and circumstances, in the absence of a mechanism of checks and balances, we end up storing erroneous and inaccurate perceptions as energy in our personal quantum fields and our Akashic Records. These self-limiting perceptions constitute our belief systems and include attitudes about our own genetic inheritance, body image, disease, sense of self-worth, and the degree to which we view ourselves, others, and the world positively, and so on. What we believe in today is what we become in the future. Beliefs are energetic patterns. It is these beliefs, not our genes, that determine what manifests as us and ultimately controls our cellular responses by influencing the way we interpret our DNA information. The experience and learned knowledge stored in our Akashic Records pervades our consciousness and drives our behavior. These are referred to as *Akashic drivers*.

Beliefs are energetic patterns. It is these beliefs, not our genes, that determine what manifests as us and ultimately controls our cellular responses by influencing the way we interpret our DNA information.

As Bruce Lipton writes, "How is the subconscious going to manage our affairs? Precisely the way it was programmed. The biggest impediments to realizing the successes of which we dream are the limitations programmed into the subconscious. These limitations not only influence our behavior, they can also play a major role in determining our physiology and our health."[8] Unfortunately, instead of learning and growing and staying in a position of neutrality with respect to what we have experienced (the experience is neither positive nor negative when we are neutral), we tend to hold on to the negative energy, and it is this energy that is stored in the subconscious mind and our Akashic Records. Unless the energy of the subconscious mind and the soul's records are cleared, unresolved issues, memories, and self-limiting perceptions continue to persist and influence us. Left unaddressed, they can impact us right down to the cellular level, ultimately creating health issues, disease, and a multitude of self-destructive behaviors including eating disorders, depression, abuse, adultery, and suicide. The quantum holographic light patterns within our personal quantum field become altered by the energy associated with these disruptive, dissonant thoughts and emotions. As the subconscious mind and our soul programs are cleared, we open ourselves up to much higher states of conscious awareness and opportunities for healing and transformation. We create much more efficient communication of the universal Source genetic code information transmitted to our DNA through our personal quantum field when the information is accurate, appropriate, and serves our highest good.

THE CONSCIOUS MIND

We must not dismiss the power of the conscious mind, however, and its ability to actively and deliberately influence the information we provide our body and our cells and to avert the potentially detrimental impact of the subconscious mind, the soul, and their programs. We have seen how our consciousness resides along with our Innate Self and Higher Self and DNA in our personal quantum field. This is the part of us that allows us to change and manipulate the information that we are transmitting to our cells and our DNA.

In addition to facilitating subconscious habitual programs, the conscious mind also has the power to be spontaneously creative in its responses to environmental stimuli. In its self-reflective capacity, the conscious mind can observe behaviors as they're being carried out. As a preprogrammed behavior is unfolding, the observing conscious mind can step in, stop the behavior, and create a new response. Thus, the conscious mind offers us free will, meaning we are not just victims of our programming.[9]

Once we realize that we are the reality and the energetic patterns we create for ourselves through our thoughts and emotions, we can begin to see the opportunity it presents for us in terms of healing. When they are negative and held statically in our personal quantum field, they manifest in the physical body, because consciousness is, in essence, a field of information that informs our DNA.

Because we are in a state of continual creation, when we resist an area of life to some degree, we manufacture experiences that reflect our resistance. But, as a deliberate creator, we can apply the basic laws that govern the physical, emotional, and mental bodies to achieve wellness. The brain imprints all suppressive thoughts, feelings, and behaviors or belief systems as habit. How we think affects our emotions, and conversely, emotions affect our mental and physical states of being. Perpetual emotional energy is captured in our personal quantum field from deeply engrained and continual thought patterns, created as a result of the ideas and perceptions we have about ourselves, others and society, from life experiences, as well as from unexpressed emotions and actions. These patterns constitute our beliefs. If they are suppressed, unrealistic, narrow-minded or self-limiting in any way, they can make us sick.

There are many psychological as well as spiritual tools and practices existing today that promote the development of self-awareness and the expansion of consciousness. Self-awareness provides us with the opportunity to know ourselves and encourages us to explore our own thoughts and emotions in a nonjudgmental and objective way, without the influence of ego or personal agenda. When we can do this, we are able to accept and love ourselves for who we are unconditionally and, from there, move toward choosing appropriate behaviors and actions that serve our highest good in all aspects of our lives, including our health and wellness. Through this process of transformation, we can shed the burden of self-limiting beliefs and perceptions to illuminate the truth of who we really are. This can have a profound effect on our state of health and the propensity with which we may manifest disease and illness through our DNA's response to the information it is being provided.

One of my practitioners taught a workshop using a simple but powerful technique to engage the conscious mind in regulating the negative impacts that thoughts and emotions have on us and our field's energy. Using a metaphor, she described our energy field as being encased in something like a fish net. The current, which is analogous to energy or life force, is supposed to flow freely and easily through the fish net. Thoughts and emotions float along in the current, flowing through the fish net. As souls, we are only meant to extract the learning that these thoughts and emotions bring to us as experience. We are not meant to hold on to these thoughts and emotions in our nets, especially those that are charged (negative or positive), as we so often do. The goal is to maintain our neutrality through conscious awareness and discernment, simply recognizing and noticing their presence, before deflecting them or letting them go. If we can expand our perspective sufficiently to recognize this dynamic, although we may not be able to control the event or triggers that create a particularly negative situation, we can control how we respond to it. It does not necessarily mean we ignore them, but we can choose not to resonate and assimilate their energy into our personal quantum field. Consciously responding with positive intent and a sense of nonjudgment, compassion, or gratitude, for example, can help maintain a more balanced energetic environment in our field, so as to avoid problems in our physical bodies down the road.

Bruce Lipton, in describing the work of Candace Pert, author of *Molecules of Emotion,* says that, "through self-consciousness, the mind can use the brain to generate 'molecules of emotion' and override the system. While proper use of consciousness can bring health to an ailing body, inappropriate unconscious control of emotions can easily make a healthy body diseased."[10]

Scientists have been investigating the impact that meditation, as a means of expanding our conscious awareness, has on the body. A recent article published in *Scientific American* on the subject indicates that meditation can rewire brain circuits to produce salutary effects not just on the mind and the brain but on the entire body. The article explains that

> some evidence even exists that meditation and its ability to enhance overall well-being may diminish inflammation and other biological stresses that occur at a molecular level. A collaborative study . . . showed that one day of intensive mindfulness practice in experienced meditators turned down the activity of inflammation-related genes and altered the functioning of enzymes involved with turning genes on and off. . . . [Another] study . . . looked at the effect of meditation on a molecule involved with regulating the longevity of a cell. The molecule in question was an enzyme called telomerase that lengthens DNA segments at the ends of chromosomes. The segments, called telomeres, ensure stability of the genetic material during cell division. They shorten every time a cell divides, and when their length decreases, below a certain critical threshold, the cell stops dividing and gradually enters a state of senescence. Compared with a control group, the meditators showed the most profound reductions in psychological stress and also had higher telomerase activity by the end of the retreat. This finding suggests that mindfulness training might slow process of cellular aging among some practitioners.[11]

Judith Kravitz, founder of a sound and breath meditation technique called Transformational Breath, says that

> . . . [I]n a meditative state, you're able to increase the breadth of the range of frequencies your brain can process, increasing your ability to access information. Accessing and processing information renders you more aware. More awareness refines your nervous system and enables you to receive information of both higher frequencies and lower frequencies. Ability to access (hear) more frequencies, raises your vibration and your awareness.[12]

Therefore, by virtue of our quantum nature, what we think and feel, consciously and unconsciously, affects our DNA and ultimately influences our genetic coding. This is critical to our understanding of the mechanisms that contribute to disease.

> **❝**
> **Therefore, by virtue of our quantum nature, what we think and feel, consciously and unconsciously, affects our DNA and ultimately influences our genetic coding. This is critical to our understanding of the mechanisms that contribute to disease.**
> **❞**

6

Consequences of DNA Misinformation

Our Causal Nature

If you want to see what your thoughts were like yesterday, look at your body today. If you want to see what your body will look like tomorrow, look at your thoughts today.

INDIAN PROVERB[1]

TRIGGERS FOR ENERGETIC DISTORTIONS IN OUR FIELD

Many people behave as though disease is caused by something in our external environment—an outside malevolent force acting upon them, rather than the internal environment they create for themselves. Based on my own experience and personal observations, allopathic medicine focuses on symptom management, offering medication and treatment options to help patients defend themselves against the assault of these perceived invisible forces. I believe this approach further entrenches this prevailing attitude about disease within our culture. We are rarely taught or realize that we can exercise options to avert illness, heal, and even eliminate disease within ourselves and that we do not necessarily have to accept its fate.

> Universe is essence . . . all creation comes out of that essence: our consciousness, mind, feelings, and physical body. Our health or disease is created by us through this process. It is us. Disease is the result of a distortion in our consciousness (our intent) that blocks the expression of our essence from coming through all the levels into the physical. Disease is an expression of how we have tried to separate ourselves from our deeper meaning . . . disease is a signature of something else. It is a signature of the underlying imbalanced energies that created it . . . the disease is a physical manifestation of a deeper disturbance.[2]

In addition to our physical bodies, our mental, emotional, and spiritual subtle energetic bodies represent our personal quantum field. The energetic patterns and imprints in these subtle bodies reflect our thoughts, attitudes, and behaviors generated as a result of the beliefs, originating in the subconscious mind and soul. These inform our DNA and shape what is known and manifested by the physical body.

> The Luminous Energy Field [personal quantum field] contains information that can kill us or heal us . . . it holds the blueprint of our body just as an architectural drawing holds the design of a house . . . but unlike a physical blueprint, which is separate and remains intact as the house ages, our luminous template is continually informed by the positive and negative incidents we experience during our lives. Unresolved psychological and spiritual traumas become engraved like scratch marks in our luminous fields. Positive experiences do not leave a mark. . . . The blueprint that shaped and molded us since we were inside our mother's womb contains the memories of our former lifetimes—the way we suffered, the way we loved, how we were ill . . . these imprints contain instructions that predispose us to repeating certain events from the past.[3]

Like the saying, "energy goes where the attention flows," if we focus on limiting beliefs, thoughts, or emotions, more energy is appropriated toward creating the lower vibrational state that these represent. Therefore, our thoughts, emotions, and spiritual state are more than just "things." If they are negative, they represent potentially lower frequencies that distort the DNA information contained in our personal quantum field and the effectiveness with which it can be communicated to our cells. We know from our understanding of quantum fields thus far that a state of coherence through higher vibrational states facilitates better information transfer. "Studies have shown that holding positive thoughts in our heart [heartspace] creates coherency between electromagnetic and bio-photon emissions [quantum genetic information] which then changes the DNA, so that our bodies are healthier. In other words, DNA can at least partly be controlled by thoughts."[4]

❝

In addition to our physical bodies, our mental, emotional, and spiritual subtle energetic bodies represent our personal quantum field. The energetic patterns and imprints in these subtle bodies reflect our thoughts, attitudes, and behaviors generated as a result of the beliefs, originating in the subconscious mind and soul. These inform our DNA and shape what is known and manifested by the physical body.

❞

Feelings such as love, joy, and gratitude are very high vibrational energies, whereas those that involve anger, sadness, and self-deprecation, for example, are lower. These lower vibrational states are expressed at the cellular level and, as previously stated, this cellular vibration determines the level of consciousness of your cells. Hypothetically, disease cannot exist at these higher vibrational levels where coherence in energetic information is present, since disease itself is seen as a lower vibration. Under such circumstances, effective information transfer needed for proper biological functioning is compromised, increasing the potential for disease. Experiments by Fritz-Albert Popp measuring the patterns of biophotons of people who were ill demonstrated that cancer patients had lost their ability to follow natural periodic biological rhythms, exhibit energetic coherence in their personal energy fields, and had too little light. Patients with multiple sclerosis showed the opposite, where they were taking in too much light, which he believed was inhibiting the ability of their cells to do their job. His findings indicate that a state of energetic balance is required to achieve a healthy state and that coherence is the middle ground between the two, somewhere between chaos and order.[5]

A multitude of factors, driven largely at the Akashic (soul) and subconscious levels as described, lend themselves to this compromised energetic environment. There are many resulting discordant thoughts and emotions generated from these two areas. Some of the more notable ones, and certainly some of the ones I experienced, are summarized below:

- Fear and resistance to change
- Unwillingness to acknowledge our own needs or desires
- Need to please others or other's needs before our own
- Inappropriate boundaries between ourselves and others
- Unworthiness, low self-esteem, and lack of self-worth
- Inability to let go of things we cannot control
- Worry and anxiety created from a lack of faith and an ability to trust
- Unwillingness to acknowledge the free will of others
- Blame and lack of forgiveness
- Manifesting disease as a means of gaining love and attention

- Manifesting disease as a means of avoiding painful or undesirable situations
- Victimhood or martyrdom
- Absence of meaning or purpose in one's life
- Taking on someone else's pain
- Desire to suffer
- Grief and loss[6]

It is the conscious thoughts and emotions resulting from experiences that we have had that shape our propensity toward disease more than anything else. As we have seen, they exist as a form of discordant energy that impacts our personal quantum field by creating distortions that represent blocks or impediments to the flow of energy, altering the integrity of Source genetic information represented as light patterns within the field and the information provided to our DNA. Therefore, we become ill when the light patterns interacting in our personal quantum fields created by these undesirable situations are quite literally out of sync or resonance.

EVIDENCE OF DISTORTION

Indications of distortion in our energetic signatures include *DNA markers,* or discordant frequencies that appear as incorrect color patterns of energy in various areas of the physical body, and *miasms,* which are energetic traces represented by vibrational patterns that remain in our personal quantum field from the past that are associated with the memory of a disease or its triggers.

DNA Markers
DNA markers anchor the light patterns that are illuminated in our personal quantum field within our physical bodies and can be observed using inner sight. Each DNA marker actually represents groups or arrays of frequencies (color). These markers are a convenient way for us to recognize the patterns that need to be changed, through the

colors they represent. If we observe a frequency other than its normal resonant frequency, meaning a discordant frequency, we know the patterns require changing.

The five major patterns that were present for me were the following:

1. Self-abandonment
2. Self-deprivation
3. Sense of separateness of self from the greater whole
4. Subjugation of others
5. Unlovable, sense of worthlessness

The core patterns associated with DNA markers are patterns of reaction that manifest early on in life, as a result of the soul programming and our life experiences, by the mechanisms described earlier. They reflect the reality that we have created for ourselves through our own beliefs about our lives and our relationships with families, friends, and those that are closest to us. The patterns reveal how we see ourselves and our lives from this distorted view through the lens of our own biased perception—our lack of self-love and acceptance or feelings of unworthiness, for example. We subconsciously adjust to the energetic imbalance these create in our fields by over- or undercompensating for the imbalance, which results in a complex weave of patterns within our personal quantum field. These discordant frequencies or DNA markers, therefore, are an indication of an alteration in the overall pattern of energy, or our true energetic signature. In order for us to be able to achieve energetic coherence and optimal health, our field must contain the appropriate frequencies represented by our inherent, harmonious energetic signature. If any are missing, incorrect, or insufficient, we may manifest disease.

I was guided to a gifted practitioner and spiritual medium who is able to see "through" the physical body as if it were transparent. During one of my treatment sessions, through her inner sight, she observed the presence of these DNA markers, each illuminated as an area or spot of a particular color of light at various locations in my body. There were five in total, each

> In order for us to be able to achieve energetic coherence and optimal health, our field must contain the appropriate frequencies represented by our inherent, harmonious energetic signature. If any are missing, incorrect, or insufficient, we may manifest disease.

correlating to one of my disease conditions along with the thought and emotional patterns associated with them (see table 1, p. 102). She explained that the colors the markers were displaying were not their correct, resonant frequency. The DNA marker related to my breast cancer, for example, was illuminated in that particular region of my body as a pale green color, yet its resonant frequency should have been represented by more of a pale green color. I was amazed that I could actually see the impact my thoughts and emotions on the energetic integrity of my personal quantum field in a tangible way. This was a very powerful visualization exercise for me.

When I inquired about these DNA markers in one of my channels, I received a vision describing the effect of the frequency anomalies on physical DNA. I was shown the typical representation of the DNA double helix with base pairs as the ribs between the two strands. In this simple visual metaphor, the frequency anomaly shines its pulsing light on the DNA, but eventually the DNA ribs or base pairs, containing the gene sequencing codes, begin to decompose as this discordant energy expresses itself. This was to indicate that gene coding is altered in this way. Some mechanism of DNA communication was also inferred in which the DNA passes this same message of transcription on to other DNA, providing instructions for them

TABLE I. DNA MARKERS—SELF PATTERN ANALYSIS

DNA Marker	Pattern Characteristics	Disease/ Condition	Thoughts/ Emotions	Correct Frequency (Color)	Altered Frequency (Color)
1	Self-deprivation	Cervical spinal deformities and issues; occipital tumor	Self-worthlessness; resignation; urgency to escape; sense of injustice; lack of joy	Purple	Red/Gray
2	Separateness	Lumbar spinal deformities and issues	Fear of external world; no sense of belongingness and wholeness; sense of being alone and abandoned	Midnight Purple	Lilac Purple
3	Lack of Self-Love	Breasts	Not lovable; cannot love others; doubt; lack of confidence; self-punishment	Emerald Green	Pale Green
4	Self-Abandonment	Thoracic spinal deformities and issues; T8 spinal tumor; iliopsoas abnormalities	Fear of self; lack of self-honor; self-denial; uncomfortable with self; self-avoidance	Blood Red Orange	Pale Orange
5	Subjugation	Hip issue; pelvic abnormalities; sacral tumor	Judgment of self and others; impatience; intolerance; inflexible; agitation; grief	White	Yellowish Green

to follow suit. When the DNA markers are removed and the associated patterns are lifted, the base pairs are repaired and there is a re-regulation of normal gene functioning.

From an energetic perspective, disease is typically indicated by an imbalance in energy or a decrease in vibration. A healthy person has a higher vibration and, therefore, an ability to retain more sound and light, which is stored in our cells and DNA.

In their healthiest state, your cells would resonate without needing to interchange many biophotons. You would expect the biophoton emissions to be coherent. If energy begins to decline and sound resonance is falling, your cells increase their communication by radiating more photons. If you become diseased your photon emissions become incoherent. Moving towards chaos, your cell is losing structure and its intercellular communication system is requesting a wide array of frequencies to rebalance itself, but it is also losing structure and giving up vibration.[7]

The incoherent photon emissions described here create the abnormal light patterns associated with these DNA markers.

It's your own multidimensional "voice" giving instructions to the quantum part of your DNA, which then results in the actual chemical changes that are occurring in the codes within your 3D genome. But now the results are going to be seen, and you can begin by removing these markers, and when you do, they stay removed. This means that something quantum you do today can change the chemistry of your gene-producing DNA so greatly that it will NOT be passed to your children.[8]

For those who have an ability to observe the human light body through inner sight or work with light frequencies, DNA markers represent a powerful tool that can be used to identify detrimental changes in the energetic field that may manifest as disease when appropriate triggers are present. The fact that these frequencies can be modified by our own consciousness through our Innate Self, without any form of physical intervention as I have shown, is equally as promising. The means by which this is achieved is described in a later chapter.

Miasms

Similar to the concept of DNA markers, energetic tendencies toward manifesting particular disease are called *miasms,* a term coined in the early days of homeopathic medicine. While we may not always manifest the disease, we carry the energy imprint, in other words, the vibrational pattern of one. According to Hahnemann, a noted homeopathy practitioner, miasms can be planetary, inherited, or acquired in the course of a person's lifetime and were deemed to be the root cause of chronic disease and a contributing factor to many acute diseases. It was thought that planetary miasms could penetrate the physical body but are stored by the collective consciousness of the planet and in the ethers (nonlocally). Inherited miasms were believed to be stored in the cellular memory of individuals, while acquired miasms were normally obtained during a person's lifetime through mechanisms such as infection or toxicity.

As Richard Gerber, author of *Vibrational Medicine,* points out, like DNA markers, miasms represent a totally different concept in the mechanism of disease causation. For example, miasms may be acquired as a result of an infectious agent, but the infection itself is not the miasm. Even though the disease-causing organism may be eradicated by antibiotic therapy, subtle energetic traces of the infectious agent may persist at an unseen level. According to his description, these disease-associated energy traces are incorporated into the individual's biomagnetic field and higher subtle bodies. The miasms reside there until their latent toxic potential is released into the molecular/cellular level of the body, where disruptive changes or diseases manifest. Miasms weaken the natural body defenses in particular areas, creating a tendency toward manifesting disease at a later time. These acquired miasms may be caused by exposure to a variety of noxious agents including bacteria, viruses, toxic chemicals, and even radiation.

Hahnemann suggests that gene coding for the expression of a disease can be passed from generation to generation undetected, via energetic pathways. Although the exact mechanism by which a condition actually manifests in the physical body deviates slightly from what has been indicated here in terms of quantum dynamics, his supposition that a miasm is not necessarily a disease but the potential for a disease that exists at an energetic level remains consistent with the idea of DNA markers. He states that "the merger of the soul's forces and ethereal properties determine when a miasm will arise in the physical body to become an active disease."[9]

ILLNESS AND DISEASE

Reasons for the development of illness and disease in the body very often cannot be reliably explained based on physical symptoms and diagnostic evidence alone, and must include consideration of emotional, mental, and spiritual, as well as environmental factors.

Diagnoses and Physical Symptoms

The majority of my diagnoses, which had thus far evaded my allopathic practitioners' attempts at testing and diagnostic imaging, came from my own intuitive inquiries, from Shamanic journeys initially, and from channeling sessions later. The information obtained from these sources was verified by exceptionally gifted health practitioners and medical intuitives, and was well correlated to my physical symptoms. Unfortunately for those with elusive and chronic disease or rare disorders, diagnosis by conventional medical means can be exceedingly difficult and sometimes nearly impossible. This is particularly true given that the technology and the means available for their detection still has limitations—laboratory testing results may fall within the normal range and diagnostic imaging may fail to show evidence of the problem. My experience suggests then, that arriving at a definitive diagnosis based on physical evidence alone may be unachievable under these circumstances, or only an educated guess based on prevailing symptoms and their correlation to specific diseases or disorders, according to existing medical knowledge or experience. Diagnosis, therefore, in the conventional medical sense is no more an exact science than the intuitive methods used to derive an understanding of what was occurring in my body, particularly when we consider the astounding capabilities that some individuals have in perceiving physical matter and nonphysical antimatter through their multisensory perception. As mentioned previously, these abilities are well documented and can be explained and substantiated from a quantum perspective, in countless cases.

Regardless, the understanding that I gained through these nonconventional means about what was happening in my body proved to be invaluable insight that assisted me in linking the diagnoses and symptoms with all of the emotional, mental, and spiritual, as well as environmental triggers. I was then able to create a complete picture of the energetic and physiological mechanisms that ultimately had culminated in the development of my illness and disease. It is doubtful that physical diagnostic evidence and test results alone would have been sufficient to put together the pieces of what had transpired at the cellular and genetic level, given the involvement of quantum fields and information described earlier. I felt an immense amount of relief in knowing there were real reasons for my terrible symptoms and failing condition. Often, when practitioners are unable to find the reason for a patient's pain and discomfort or for their perplexing symptoms, patients are left with the impression "it is all in their head." Once I understood what I was feeling and experiencing was indeed real, no matter how dire the circumstances were, I was able to release the burden of self-blame and guilt I'd taken on as a result of inaccurate diagnoses. Healing began in earnest after these important revelations, once the uncertainty that something was indeed wrong was eliminated.

A myriad of physical symptoms accompanied the various maladies, all of which contributed to the extreme difficulty I experienced in coping and maintaining some semblance of comfort and mobility along the way. General symptoms included the following:

- overwhelming feeling of malaise
- weight loss
- extreme fatigue
- fever and chills
- brain fog

- vision changes
- insomnia
- digestive changes
- acid reflux and abdominal pain
- adrenal fatigue and low cortisol levels
- swollen glands

In addition to the pain I was already experiencing as a result of the degenerative changes to my spine (disc herniation, fusing, nerve damage, and impingement and post-radiation changes of the thoracic spine), other major symptoms included the following:

- breast tenderness and pain
- lymph node (armpit) pain
- jaw pain
- spinal pain, pressure, and stiffness
- hip and sacroiliac joint pain and immobility
- pelvic pain
- bladder and bowel discomfort and dysfunction
- ear drainage difficulties, tinnitus, and vertigo
- shoulder pain, inflammation, and immobility
- vascular changes in mid back, hands, and feet
- general muscle ache and joint pain, headaches, metallic taste in mouth

Emotional, Mental, and Spiritual Factors

Upon reflection, it became clear to me how my emotional and mental state had created the blocks and dysfunctional patterns my practitioners described as being present in my personal quantum field. These had undoubtedly contributed to what had manifested in my physical body. Initially, I felt very bad about this, thinking that I'd unknowingly caused my own problems directly as a result of my behavior and actions. Once I understood there was a connection, I thought everything that had happened to me, including pain and disease, was my fault. Admittedly, how we consciously choose to think, feel, and act is a major contributing factor in what we manifest in our bodies and our lives. However, I also began to understand the significant contribution that the subconscious mind and soul and our divine plan make to what plays out for us in our lives—the people and experiences we attract in order to learn the lessons our souls require, and the energetic residue that remains if our Akashic Records are not cleared that can drive things in a direction that does not necessarily serve our highest good. These feelings began to ease when, early in my healing journey, I received a reading from a spiritual medium that was profound and pivotal in my understanding of myself and the challenges I had experienced throughout my life. Many of my issues stemmed from the past and from energy and beliefs stored at the subconscious mind and soul level that, until this point, I was completely unaware. I became reassured by the fact that, with my own permission, a healthy dose of self-love, and with the help of Spirit, Innate, and Higher Self, the discordant energy that these circumstances had created could be rectified and the subconscious and Akashic drivers dismantled in order to heal. It felt good to know that the damage was not permanent.

Despite my functionality on so many levels in my life, and how some might have perceived me on the surface, I felt a real and palpable sense of fear at a very deep internal level. I was afraid of failing. I was afraid of the future and of what I did not know. I was afraid of taking risks and of being judged. I learned from the reading that my thoughts and emotions were pervaded by this sense of internal insecurity and sense of my own wrongness. Although these were rooted in past lives (and thus the energy stored in my Akashic Record), there were certain circumstances that I found stressful in my current life that reinforced these feelings. These included some continual challenges I had experienced in relationships with partners and family members over the years. I had little confidence in trusting my own instincts nor in my ability to listen and respond to my own internal voice of reason or to think independently.

Sometimes, I found myself lost in a conflicted mental state and scared of my own thinking. Life seemed to become more difficult as I aged, until I eventually gave in to this fear and insecurity. Somehow I came to believe my thoughts and feelings were wrong and inappropriate. My life seemed precarious and tenuous, and I felt isolated and alone. I was worried that whatever I said or did would not be accepted by others. I stepped outside my own self to protect myself from the painful feelings that this self-doubt had created.

I had spent years resisting the conflict I felt raging within and was influenced too much by the outside in, instead of the other way around. There was an intense side to me, a "warrior energy" that I possessed that I did not want to admit, thinking it was a bad thing instead of something that could benefit me if it was appropriately channeled. Without a place of refuge or a means of developing appropriate out-lets for this energy, I tended to sabotage myself and my relationships with others. I became defensive and tended to take things personally. I struggled to make sense of my relationships and interactions, feeling very misunderstood.

I felt bad and was confused about my goals and purpose in life as well as my relationships with others. I was constantly apologizing to others when I felt a need to honor myself and my needs. Again, there were past-life origins for these feelings associated with my inability to take care of myself. I had placed greater importance on taking care of everything and everyone else around me. I had become my own worst critic, and I certainly did not need anyone else to help me with that— I could not forgive myself for not asserting myself.

I had experienced a lot of inner turmoil around my own ability to love and honor myself over many years, which worsened as I grew older. I found it difficult to receive nurturing when it was offered, particu-larly when I did not feel loved or important to anybody else, including my own family. I felt I simply could not surrender and be vulnerable to whatever or whomever was in my life at the time. What I hadn't realized until that point was how much unhappiness I had created for myself when I was not true to my needs, wants, or feelings. I could not let go and surrender to the process of healing and be open to whatever experiences my life would bring. I was judging myself and, in doing so, I had abandoned myself.

I moved on to regular treatment sessions with a natural healing arts practitioner and shaman as a means of addressing my issues. By that point, I was quite ill and was experiencing a great deal of pain and discomfort. I recall her saying, "I can guarantee that we can heal and resolve your issues at the emotional, mental, and spiritual levels, but to do so at the physical level is much harder." We spent several years working very intently in these areas, clearing and balancing my energy and doing soul work.

The resistance to letting go revealed itself in the form of incredible muscle tension and inability to relax, which contributed greatly to my pain and discomfort. I held a rigidity that literally trapped patterns of energy close to the surface of my body, underneath my skin. As this continued, I found myself developing a propensity toward seriousness. Sadness, anger, grief, and loss welled up inside me creating a block to the energy flow throughout my body. My life force was drained, and I told her I was emotionally, mentally, and physically exhausted trying to hold myself together. She observed my soul hovering quite happily outside my body, and quite frankly I thought to myself: who could blame it for not wanting to get back in a body that felt like this? I struggled to find any joyful or happy moments. My suffering only isolated me further.

Shamanic journeys and soul work revealed that I had soul programs (referred to as *soul contracts* in Shamanic practices) that were creating significant problems for me. Somewhere along the way, I had adopted an intense desire to suffer as though my soul was doing penance for some wrongful deed in the past. Another one showed how, at a soul level, I had registered everything anyone had ever thought about me and how they perceived me. I had actually allowed others to define me through their judgments.

The uncertainty, insecurity, and fear I had felt for so many years had eventually eroded my energetic integrity and, when coupled with some environmental triggers including the toxicity, had now manifested in the physical body as a cancerous jaw tumor. As the tumor was being cleared through the application of light and spiritual healing energy, a spiritual guide with whom my practitioner works advised me that the tumor was related to fear. There had been past-life trauma in which I had been persecuted for speaking out about certain spiritual and religious truths. It comes as no surprise that this area of the body correlates to the third chakra in the subtle energy body, which is associated with communication, speaking truths, and exerting self-will. As recipient of my very first spiritual healing, I was absolutely astonished that something as potentially grave and physical as a cancerous jaw tumor could simply disappear in the span of about twenty minutes with the administering of light energy directed through the hands of my practitioner. I felt truly humbled that Spirit had deemed me to be worthy of such a benevolent gift.

Throughout this whole ordeal, I had experienced a lot of difficulty in my relationship with my partner. We had repeated altercations that left me feeling wounded and victimized. I was disillusioned by his lack of attentiveness and inability to offer me any physical or emotional comfort, particularly given my recent physical challenges. He was playing out soul programs of his own that centered on patterns of self-righteousness and blame. Even though I recognized that these were not mine, I felt powerless to avoid their perilous influence on my perpetual lack of self-esteem and ever present self-doubt. I limited myself by second guessing the opportunities that lay ahead of me. I was the opposite of him. Under the circumstances, these feelings eroded my confidence immeasurably, cementing my own patterns more permanently. My defensive response was an outward projection of my frustration and anger. For the longest time, I could not find a way to recognize the triggers and let them go. It took me quite a while to recognize that whether right or wrong, indignation is futile and that I needed to find ways to dissipate the intensity of these emotions. Unfortunately, by that time, the impact this already had on my energy and state of health was readily apparent.

Many of the problems I had experienced in my sacral and lumbar spine were related to emotional issues during my childhood surrounding sexuality (inability to feel deep love and connection) and my identity (meaning and purpose in life). These manifested in part as the nerve problems I was experiencing. As an eight year old, I felt misunderstood by my parents. I knew I was different in some way, even then. I could not be the person I knew I was meant to be. It was like the invisible world (Spirit) was following me around, but I could not access it. On the outside, I knew I could be strong, articulate, and confident, but on the inside, it was an entirely different story. Additional treatments eventually revealed that the ruminations and almost obsessive thoughts I had been experiencing over the last year or so related to inconsistencies or gaps in the flow of energy in my spine. Once again, I was reminded of just how pervasive our thoughts and emotions can be on what manifests for us energetically and physically.

I underwent an aggressive detoxification program to help rid my body of the heavy metals and toxins, including those assumed to be associated with some of the injections I had received as treatments in the past few years. It had left my body systems compromised and my immunity and overall constitution weakened, resulting in the return of the cancer to some soft tissue areas around my jaw. Fortunately, through a very powerful treatment of light, it was once again laid to rest. Much like the DNA markers, the discordant frequency was shown as a light blue color, which, when transformed to its true resonant frequency, showed up as a dark blue color when the healing was completed. During the healing, however, I was once again reminded by spiritual beings through my practitioner to be aware of the thoughts and feelings I was holding inside and how it contributed to the reality I was creating for myself. This was an important teaching, and one I took seriously as an opportunity to learn about myself, rather than as a criticism. I did not feel shame as though I had been harshly admonished. Instead, I was grateful that this had been pointed out to me, and I knew that by applying a little more self-awareness, it was within my power to step out of these old and negative patterns.

Several months later, I experienced a major breakthrough and was offered a healing for my hip dysfunction. My practitioner had observed the presence of a synovial-type lesion about 2 inches in length, recessed in behind the femoral head in my left hip cavity that had evaded detection during the MRI. This, in addition to a small bone chip (osteophyte) on top of the femoral head and the abnormal positioning of my pelvis, had resulted in the debilitating pain and difficulties I had been experiencing for many years. This came as welcome news, since at that time surgery was not considered justifiable by my doctors, based on their understanding of my case and the lack of diagnostic evidence from their perspective. During the healing, a physiological imprint of the hip and its surrounding muscles, tendons, and ligaments, going back to when I was ten years old, was brought forward into present time and reintroduced into my physical and energetic body. I was awestruck at the unbounded potential that exists for healing even severe and long-standing physical abnormalities through energetic and spiritual means. I felt hopeful about the future for the first time in years, and my resolve to continue my journey was notably strengthened. In the aftermath of my hip healing, I came to understand just how much emotional drain had occurred in living with the burden of the significant physical compromise and difficulty that the hip problem had represented for me. I also learned that it had been associated with the emotion of grief. The death of my identical twin at birth (stillbirth) and soul-related factors were the main drivers for this emotion.

The retrieval of my soul during one of my treatments marked another major turning point for me. I was finally able to put behind me the life-long, distant feelings that something had always been missing, that I had felt some kind of inexplicable loss, sadness, and abandonment. A very vital piece of me had come home. I realized then how unsettled and incomplete I had felt prior to this and how critical soul work is in reconstituting our wholeness as a part of our healing. I felt significantly better afterward—more like myself than perhaps I'd ever been. A week later, I experienced a powerful release of anger, along with my tendencies toward ruminating and constant negative thought patterns.

However, the battle continued to rage on within and, despite repeated efforts by my practitioner at a very deep level, I was still resisting embodying some of the resonant vibrations that were being introduced to me through the treatments. Although I had come to terms with some of the reasons for my discord and their effects, I struggled to let go and forgive myself. The ultimate source of this resistance was not revealed until sometime later in the course of my healing. My energy meridians during Chinese Five Element treatments reflected that I still had a difficult time expelling what was bad for me and what did not serve me. When it became apparent that the next challenge, breast cancer, was upon me, I had almost given up. At a very deep level, a part of me could not decide whether it wanted to stay alive or not. Any remaining anger and frustration had now yielded to complete despondency. Although it did not last, at the time I felt terribly discouraged and disheartened.

Although there were certainly some rather phenomenal healing events, including the healing of my hip, the eradication of the cancer in my jaw area, and the fact that I had regained a great deal of life force and energetic balance, I still experienced a lot of symptoms and did not feel well. Along with this, I had also experienced very rapid expansion in my own personal spiritual growth and capacity. Just as I thought I was moving toward opportunities for more extensive and possibly complete healing, there was a major shift, and I was guided away from this approach. I had poured all my efforts into learning about disease and healing from a holistic perspective, developing skills as a holistic practitioner and intuitive, and now it seemed the remaining physical ailments (and ones I had but was not aware of at the time) were to be understood and addressed in another way. I wrestled down the fear of uncertainty and did my best to move forward, despite the fact I had no idea what the future had in store for me.

Following this, I moved on to another practitioner. In the beginning, she focused a great deal on finding ways to support me through energetic and physical application of supplements and remedies to support my extremely depleted physical state. As we continued our work together, many soul programs were cleared that were at the root of my remaining physical challenges and difficulties. The tumors she discovered on my lower sacral spine and in the occipital region of my head were related to soul programs that had instilled a desire to suffer, feelings of failure, abandonment, hate, doubt, and guilt in me. Once these programs were cleared, they simply vanished and all symptoms associated with them disappeared within a few hours. Through her, five specific soul patterns associated with the DNA markers in my body were also removed. By that time, I had also separated my right shoulder as a result of a bike accident and was experiencing a lot of pain and discomfort in that area of my body. This turned out to be associated with a soul program related to unworthiness. Chronic insomnia had plagued me most of my life, from early childhood on. My sleep quality improved once a few soul programs were cleared involving past lives where I was subjected to constant danger and had a need to "sleep with one eye open," along with some frequency adjustments made to my pineal gland. Soul programs relating to pelvic pain I had experienced since my early teens were also cleared, once again resulting in a significant reduction in symptoms in this area. I began to move into a more calm and centered way of being. I was more responsive to whatever came up, as opposed to being reactive—challenges seemed more like small hurdles instead of big insurmountable walls that I had to get myself over. As I relaxed and let go of any fear about my remaining symptoms—what might still be wrong with me or what was going to happen—the pain and discomfort began to dissipate.

There were many other extremely deep and equally profound adjustments made to my light body and physical body during the course of these treatments. Many of the changes occurred as a result of my own efforts as my conscious awareness deepened, my spiritual practice intensified, and I dedicated myself to the journey inward, to a place of deeper meaning and purpose. Although they also had a significant impact on my healing and transformation, they are not covered here as part of the subject of this book. Many of these were to facilitate an expansion in my consciousness and spiritual evolution, promote my ability to translate, modify, and assimilate specific light frequencies, and to expand my capabilities and receptivity in receiving multidimensional information at new levels. They have opened up whole new dimensions of consciousness and areas of exploration to me for continued and future work in the area of consciousness and DNA and have enabled me to move from the role of patient to practitioner. My path undoubtedly fits the wounded-healer archetype, and many of the things I learned, as well as the way in which I healed, have become useful in my ability to serve others with similar issues and challenges.

Environmental Factors

It became apparent that, in my case, oxidative stress resulting from three sources—free radicals associated with radiation treatment to the tumor in my thoracic spine; untreated toxicity; and the physical injuries I had sustained over the years—were the main culprits in triggering the development of the various disease states, given my compromised energetic state due to the mental, emotional, and spiritual factors described. Oxidative stress produces reactive oxygen species (chemically reactive molecular species containing oxygen) that can affect our ability to detoxify the reactive intermediates, namely, free radicals, which are very prevalent in disease states. In all likelihood, the oxidative stress had eventually, through mechanisms that will be described in subsequent chapters, created a chronic and severe condition of inflammation in my body and had also contributed to the tumors and cancer.

I had undergone a thirty-day stretch of radiation treatment for a very rare kind of noncancerous tumor that had occupied a significant portion of one of the vertebra in my thoracic spine. It is well known that radiation exposure creates free radicals, one of the reactive oxygen species involved here. A few years later, test results revealed that I had abnormally high levels of aluminum, mercury, and lead concentrations in my body, likely owing to exposure during my time as a petroleum laboratory technician analyzing for heavy metals in samples, many years prior. This work also involved working extensively with organic solvents and other chemicals, many of which are extremely harmful and carcinogenic when normal exposure limits are exceeded. The test results also indicated abnormally high levels of a number of organic solvents and compounds. Toxins can disrupt the electrical potential of the cell membranes and mitochondria as well as deactivate electron transfer and disturb oxygen-dependent energy production. Toxic overload also creates acid reactions in the body, making energy production at the cellular level inefficient when less oxygen is utilized and less energy is produced. It was hard to suppress my dismay given that it had taken over nineteen years since the initial exposure to harmful substances and six years since the radiation treatment for the effects to be identified and more fully understood, particularly through my seemingly unorthodox means of inquiry. In addition, I had injured my hip and shoulder, in separate biking accidents. A disparity of oxygen and acidic conditions were also prevalent where injured, necrotic tissue existed. Clearly, the path to destruction in my own physical body had been laid a very long time ago. Despite the sobering discovery, I was feeling a little less stressed now that the whole picture was coming together.

These environmental triggers, when coupled with the emotional, mental, and spiritual factors previously described, had a tremendous impact on my cell and genetic response and, thus, the manifestation of physiological impairment and disease. Details of these mechanisms will be described in detail in the next chapter.

7

Physical Responses to Energetic Information

Energetic Mechanisms

*Disease is . . . not something local, not an affectation of the
parts, but it is the state of being of the whole person at the time.*

RAJAN SANKARAN[1]

ENERGY AFFECTS PHYSIOLOGY

Electromagnetic conditions created in one's personal quantum field
influence our susceptibility to the environmental factors described in
the previous chapter. Under suboptimal conditions when that field
energy is compromised, the quantum genetic information transmitted
through the field as light is not properly modulated. This degrades the
quality and accuracy of the information received and transmitted by
our quantum DNA to our biological DNA instruction sets and creates
the corresponding dysfunction at the cellular and genetic level based on
this information. When the energetic properties of our cells are altered
in this manner, we become far more vulnerable to any detrimental
external effects that may pose a threat to normal cellular health and

immunity such as toxins, trauma, infection, or similar stresses, as well as any genetic propensity to inherited disease.

Bruce Lipton believes the cell is a "programmable chip" whose biological behavior and gene activity are controlled by environmental signals, not genes. He explains the role of integral membrane proteins (IMPs), known as receptors and effectors, in this process. Receptor proteins function as molecular "nano-antennas" located inside and outside the cells that are tuned to respond to certain environmental signals in the form of energy. The cells change shape from an inactive to an active configuration, depending on the electrical charge, creating what is known as an effector protein. He refers to this receptor/effector combination as the "fundamental units of cellular intelligence" or "units of perception" because they operate dynamically by responding to the energetic stimulus that is outside themselves, not by their genetic coding. The effector proteins respond to the incoming signal, interpret the information, and instigate a biological cellular response. These IMPs or their by-products provide signals that control the binding of the chromosome's regulatory proteins that form a sleeve around the DNA, and the "reading" of the genes so that worn-out proteins can be replaced or new proteins can be created.[2] This means, according to Lipton, that genes themselves do not control their own activity, but rather, the receptor-effector mechanism does in response to the energetic environmental signals it receives.

In his article "The Electrical Properties of Cancer Cells," Dr. Steve Haltiwanger describes how these cell receptors are activated by electrical fields via vibrational resonance, when the frequencies and amplitudes are correct. He says, "electrical oscillations can alter the electrical charge distribution in cell receptors causing the receptors to undergo conformational change just as if the receptor was activated by a chemical signal."[3] The oscillation of the electrical field affects cell receptors that respond by switching back and forth between conformations; this then turns on the activity of membrane-embedded enzymes that trigger specific cellular metabolic processes.

Each molecule has its own signature frequency, its receptor or molecule with the matching spectrum of features would tune in to this frequency. . . . They get in resonance—the vibration of one body is reinforced by the vibration of another at or near its frequency. As these two molecules resonate on the same wavelength, they would then begin to resonate with the next molecules in the biochemical chain, thus creating . . . a "cascade" of electromagnetic impulses travelling at the speed of light. This, rather than accidental collision would better explain how you initiate a virtually instantaneous chain reaction in biochemistry.[4]

Ross Adey's medical science research also confirms that the application of weak electromagnetic fields of certain windows of frequency and intensity act as first messengers to the cells by activating receptors in the cell membrane. His work supports Lipton's and Haltiwanger's theories and suggests that this electrical property of cell receptor-membrane complexes allows cells to scan incoming frequencies and tune their circuitry to allow them to resonate at particular frequencies. Adey has reported that certain frequency bands have been found to promote cancers, while others alter cell protein synthesis, DNA replication function, immune responses, and intercellular communication.[5]

Therefore, it is clear that when electromagnetic conditions in a person's personal quantum field are compromised and the frequencies are abnormal, physiologic responses at the cellular level may be adversely affected.

ENERGETIC MECHANISMS

Sondra Barrett, a recognized academic and proponent of mind-body medicine and author of *Secrets of Your Cells: Discovering Your Body's Inner Intelligence,* looks at our cells from both a scientific and a sacred perspective. She describes how the intelligent messages our cells receive are processed by the cell's basic structure, the cytoskeleton. The cytoskeleton, or cellular matrix, is comprised of the transmembrane proteins that "serve as mechanical scaffolds that organize enzymes and water and anchor the cell to structures in the extracellular matrix via linkages through the cell membrane."[6] Like Haltiwanger and Lipton, she also believes that the cell's structure is a function of the intelligence contained in its external environment. Barrett says the scaffolding connects all parts of the cell and prevents the cell from collapsing on itself. She maintains that while our external receptors may be the receivers of the messages, it is the cytoskeleton, which comprises the fabric or strings of our cells, that generates the actual cell response to the instructions received. Therefore, it is the receptors and the cytoskeleton working together that embody this intelligence.[7]

Barrett suggests that the cytoskeletal fabric is made of organized proteins that are shaped like microtubules and microfilaments. These structures respond to stimuli by changing shape or tension—and by vibrating. She notes that scientific research has shown that changes in tension affect genetic expression, and concludes that alterations in the physical state of cells can indeed alter genes. Even though cells contain the same genetic information, they seem to be able to manifest different abilities and genetic programs. In addition, Barrett also says that cells can actually see through orifices called "centrioles" and can detect infrared energy generated from neighboring cells. This provides evidence that they recognize each other energetically. Another theory has been developed that suggests "centrioles transmit information by changing their shape as a result of electrons flowing (electricity or light) from one end of the tube to the other. According to these scientists, the electron flow down our cell tubes is consciousness."[8] In other words, in this context, consciousness is light (quantum information).

Given the mechanisms by which light information is transmitted in quantum fields as electrical impulses through filaments at the macrocosm level previously described, there are some important parallels seen at the cellular level, again demonstrating the macrocosm/ microcosm holographic concept. In a similar vein to Barrett, Hameroff and others have said that the microtubules in cells create the basic structure of the cells such that they can be described as "light pipes" through which disordered wave signals transform into coherent waves that are pulsed through the rest of the body.[9] He suggests that once coherence is achieved, the photons of light can travel along these light pipes as though they were transparent, penetrating other microtubules and communicating with other photons.[10] These cytoskeletal filaments function like fiber-optic cables and electronic semiconductors in an integrated network or continuum. Cytoskeletal proteins structurally and electronically link the cell membrane with cell organelles. Therefore, every part of the body is bioelectrically linked to every other part in this way.[11] This would provide an obvious explanation for the instantaneous communication and coordination functions we see among cells in response to the light information provided to them via our quantum DNA.

The cytoskeleton then, is like a network or latticelike electrical matrix that transmits quantum genetic information as light. The carrier for the light information is acoustic waves, generated as a result of natural harmonic oscillation or vibratory conditions prevalent throughout cells and our bodies. Thus, our cells and DNA truly are the vehicles for the connection between what lies within our physical bodies and our personal quantum fields. This observation is borne out by research that indicates the following:

> DNA, in fact produces its creative effects by acting as a holographic projector of acoustic and EM [electromagnetic] information. DNA's electromagnetic and acoustic data . . . "contains the informational quintessence of the [human] hologram . . . the holographic concept of genetic expression that results in precipitated reality . . . operates using photons and phonons. . . . Superposed coherent waves of different types in the cells interact to form diffraction patterns, firstly in the acoustic domain, secondly in the electromagnetic domain." The resulting manifestation is a "quantum hologram—a translation process between acoustical and optical hologram." . . . In this way,

DNA communications can have long-term transformative effect on the whole person.[12]

In my particular case, according to my channels, a degradation in personal quantum field energy had created unstable and insufficient electrical flow (quantum holographic light information) through my body, thereby weakening the magnetic field generated as a result of the electrical flow. Normally, moving electrical charges create a magnetic field that is perpendicular (at right angles, or 90 degrees) to the flow of the charges. However, under these abnormal circumstances, there was too much offset in the angles between the two, and the electrical signal was interrupted. The mechanism was shown to me as a narrowing or a thickening in the band of light incident on the surface of the cells, indicative of the inconsistency in the electrical signal. The light appeared stagnant in some places and as thinner or thicker bands in other areas, so that when the light reached the surface of the cells, its pattern was not extended evenly on the surface of the cell. Thus, it had weakened in intensity, was incoherent, and was represented by a much narrower range of frequencies than was necessary for normal cell functioning.

Cells normally have the ability to accumulate and store charges from these electrical impulses as an electric field, which is a property known as *capacitance*. However, the generally poor energetic environment compromised the electrical flow and eventually created a condition of suboptimal capacitance associated with these incomplete (parsed) and weak electrical signals. Cells are made of materials that make them dielectric. In other words, there are no free charges so they function as insulators. This characteristic enables them to possess both conductive and capacitive capabilities so that they can transmit electrical flow without transferring energy. In the presence of an electrical field, the negatively charged ions separate from positively charged ions, located on either side of the cell membrane. With this separation, referred to as *polarization,* cells acquire an electric dipole moment.[13] Electric dipoles are essentially transducers, which means they possess a dual energetic function in which they are able to convert electrical waves into acoustic waves and vice versa. This enables them to oscillate and resonate with other cells they interact with, a characteristic known as *dielectric resonance*. When a cell acts as a dielectric resonator, it produces an electrical field around itself that is capable of interacting with similar systems.[14] When the external electrical field that is imposed is of the correct frequency and amplitude, it can create a preferential alignment of its dipoles, which is the mechanism by which electrical fields alter cell membrane structure and consequently cellular function, through the receptor/effector mechanisms described earlier.[15] This is thought to occur since cell membranes contain many dipole molecules. Conversely, when the frequency and amplitude is incorrect, corresponding cell structure and function is compromised.

CELLULAR RESPONSE

More specifically, my channels were indicating that transmembrane cell proteins that make up the cytoskeleton had been adversely affected as a result of the altered electrical signals in the body. These proteins are responsible for the transport of nutrients and waste materials between the inside and outside of the cell, as well as intracellular communication through cell signaling. They consist of linear chains made of amino acids that fold into three-dimensional shapes known as *conformational states,* depending on the prevalent electrical conditions. Under conditions of cellular stress and particularly when the electrical potential of the cell's membrane becomes more electronegative, the protein backbone structure collapses and the cellular membrane degrades. This changes their structural orientation and conformational status, resulting in a corresponding change in cellular function, as the surface receptor sites became altered in the process. Extracellular signaling molecules such as hormones, neurotransmitters (substances that carry, boost, and modulate signals between neurons and other cells in the body), as well as cytokines (small proteins secreted by cells that play a role in inflammation) that normally attach to the surface receptor sites cannot do so under these conditions. In the absence of appropriate surface receptor binding, enzymes that normally function as electrical switches to stop and start metabolic reactions occurring in cells are not released to assist in mediating a response to pain, inflammation, or abnormal cell growth and proliferation.

Positively charged mineral ions including calcium, sodium, potassium, and magnesium are normally maintained in different concentrations on either side of the cell membrane to create the cell membrane potential, which is an electrochemical force or gradient generated across the membrane. Among other things, it helps control cell membrane permeability. Changes in the transmembrane protein shape, which is essentially a change in cell membrane structure due to poor electrical conditions, also affects the transport of these ions through ion channels, closing the channels and inhibiting their passage through the cell membrane. "Healthy cells maintain inside of themselves a high concentration of potassium and a low concentration of sodium. But, when cells are injured or cancerous, sodium and water flows into the cells and potassium, magnesium, calcium, and zinc are lost from the cell interior. Then the cell membrane potential falls."[16] If too much sodium gets inside to the mitochondria, the cellular energy production begins to use sodium, but it does not work as efficiently. The waste salts become sodium salts, which are more acidic than the normal potassium salts. These acidic conditions mean that energy production becomes less efficient because less oxygen and less energy is produced as a result.[17] Disease processes ensue as a result of the intracellular communication breakdown and metabolic abnormalities created with these low membrane potentials.

Dr. Haltiwanger says that the electrical properties of tissues are related to electron availability, tissue acidity, and degree of tissue hypoxia (lack of oxygen). Apparently, the ability of the cell proteins to stay in their proper shape (conformational structure) depends on the cell being free from chemical, physical, or hypoxic damage. So, when this type of damage occurs, many cell proteins will change to an abnormal or altered state.[18] It has been reported that tissues of the body that are injured or diseased have a higher electrical resistance than the surrounding tissue. This causes electrical currents flowing through the body to avoid these areas of high resistance.[19] This most certainly was true in my case as all three of these factors figured prominently as environmental triggers in this scenario: chemical damage from toxicity, physical damage from physical injury, and hypoxic damage (oxidative stress) from radiation exposure. Dr. Haltiwanger notes that oxidative stress deactivates energy transfer and disturbs oxygen-dependent energy production in the body at the cellular level. Cellular membrane–bound organelles, known as mitochondria, responsible for generating biochemical energy (ATP) become compromised and free radicals (uncharged molecules) are produced as a by-product of mitochondrial inefficiency. The presence of free radicals induces mitochondrial membrane permeability and, thus, the cellular structures are damaged. Molecular substances normally contained within the mitochondria leak into the cytoplasm. Cytoplasmic pattern recognition receptors (PRP) recognize the leaked substances as a potential threat and form a complex called the inflammasome that activates inflammatory cytokines that recruit components of the immune system to destroy the infected cell.[20]

When cell membranes are damaged by free radicals, their ability to hold an electrical charge is disrupted along with their ability to transport minerals and other nutrients. When mitochondria are damaged by free radicals, cellular ability to make energy is impaired. When free radicals damage genetic codes, attacked cells cannot reproduce normally. Free radicals also cause lipid peroxidation [oxidative degradation] which can . . . cause damage to cell membranes lining your blood vessels. When these delicate membranes are damaged, an inflammatory process may result which leads to thickening of blood vessels with the production of arterial plaque. These tissue reactions created by free radicals are also thought to be involved in . . . the development of cancer . . . arthritis, immune disorders, and other degenerative diseases.[21]

Normally, most of the calcium stored in the cell resides in the cellular membrane structure, except during cell signaling, when some of the calcium is released and takes up temporary residence in the mitochondria. If the equilibrium balance of calcium is not maintained because cellular transport mechanisms are impaired due to the reasons cited above, a process of calcium-induced apoptosis (programmed cell death) occurs. As a result, the release of small amounts of cytochrome C protein leads to an interaction with cell receptors that causes calcium release from the cell's membrane structure. The overall increase in calcium triggers a massive release of cytochrome C, which then acts in the positive feedback loop to maintain the calcium release process through the cell receptors. In this way, this calcium can actually reach cytotoxic levels. Cytochrome C release in turn activates a number of enzymes that are responsible for destroying the cell from within.[22]

When stressful conditions imposed on the cell membrane structure are prolonged, the cell initiates a defensive process, called an "unfolded protein response." This is aimed at safeguarding cellular survival, but will initiate apoptosis and elimination of the faulty cell under extreme stress conditions. Thus the initial signal, which is the accumulation of misfolded proteins inside the cellular membrane structure, is transmitted across the cell membrane, through the cytoplasm, and into the nucleus where alterations in gene expression patterns occur. In the development of cancer and tumors, when cell stresses such as those described here are prevalent, the body's ability to rid itself of damaged cells via the process of apoptosis is compromised. In the presence of activated oncogenes (cancer-causing genes), faulty cells designated for apoptosis survive and proliferate instead.[23]

Studies have reported that the electrical potential of cancer cell membranes is significantly less than the membrane potential of healthy cells, and electrical connections are disrupted. As indicated, a reduction in electrical field strength causes degradation in the cellular membrane structure as well as alterations in the metabolic functions of the cell.[24] Degenerative changes in the surface membrane cause cells to become more permeable to water-soluble substances. Thus, an imbalance in cellular components is created, where the intracellular concentrations of sodium is high and the potassium is low as it migrates to the outside of the cell along with magnesium and calcium. As a result, these cells tend to retain more water and have a different geometry than normal cells, which in turn disrupts normal cell signaling mechanisms.[25] Degenerative changes in the inner membrane of the mitochondria cause the loss of critical mitochondrial enzymes and the overall number of mitochondria in cancer cells is reduced.[26]

Normal cells are well organized in their growth and relationships with other normal cells and stop growing at the right time. In contrast, "cancer cells are more easily detached and fail to exhibit contact inhibition of their growth. Cancer cells become estranged from normal tissue. They become bioelectrically and biochemically self-sustaining. Tissue and intercellular signaling is diminished. Growth control mechanisms fall away."[27] Essentially, cancer cells are cells that have become independent of the electrical field pattern of the body. They are withdrawn and are operating with complete disregard for their relationship to the whole organism. When this action is observed in nature—when organisms exist outside the universal pattern of creation—destruction occurs.[28]

Therefore, it is evident that my cancer, the tumors, cytotoxicity, and some of the inflammation developed and the associated disease mechanisms were sustained in these ways. The discordant energy in my personal quantum field, along with the environmental triggers, had most definitely manifested itself physiologically as cellular breakdown and dysfunction, ultimately leading to my health issues and disease conditions. I was very excited when I discovered the critically important link between our energetic and external environment and how their effects manifest themselves in the physical body. Some have certainly intimated that this is most likely the case, but I had never been able to piece the whole picture together in such a comprehensive way. Now the principles of conventional and holistic medicine had merged to my satisfaction.

Truly, as my case indicates, these aspects cannot be viewed in isolation of each other if disease is to be completely understood and addressed. If I could fully describe my situation now from a more complete perspective, I wondered, how might this important realization help others who are critically ill and struggling with the same things I had been? The possibilities seemed enormous to me.

GENETIC RESPONSE

In the same manner that an electronegative charge on the surface of the cell, characterized by an abnormally low membrane potential, is the root cause of cellular dysfunction causing disease, genetic changes can also result from the development of cellular electrical abnormalities. This is an obvious contradiction to the commonly held belief that genetic variation (mutation) is the leading cause of disease.[29] Genetic changes may include "DNA strand breaks, acquired dysfunction of DNA repair mechanisms, mutations in genes that drive cells to divide, mutations in genes that suppress cell division, and failure to properly code mRNA [correct genetic coding sequences for replication]."[30]

> **In the same manner that an electronegative charge on the surface of the cell, characterized by an abnormally low membrane potential, is the root cause of cellular dysfunction causing disease, genetic changes can also result from the development of cellular electrical abnormalities.**

Under normal conditions, genetic response, which is an ability to translate the energetic information our DNA receives (as light and sound information), is thought to be affected by our electromagnetic field as follows:

> The electrical charges stored in the cell membrane (as capacitance) are normally transferred to DNA and are involved in DNA activation. This helps create an electrical field around the genome. . . . Dr. Garnett has theorized that an alternating current oscillating circuit exists inside of cells between the cell membrane and the DNA that is conducted over electronic protein polymers. This circuit is activated during cell differentiation to trigger the expression of genes.[31]

In other words, the storage of electrical charge in the cellular membrane and the resulting electrical field that is created allows the cytoskeletons to "plug into this field and power up cell structures such as genetic material."[32] As indicated previously, DNA is coiled around protein structures in such a way as to create an inductance coil or circuit that is capable of transmitting electrical flow through its helically shaped structure. It is thought that inward electrical current flows from the cell membrane to DNA and outward current flows back from the DNA along the cytoskeletal structure or cellular matrices. From here, the energy passes through the cell membrane to the extracellular matrix (ECM).[33] This creates a pulse (alternating current oscillating circuit) within the DNA that allows it to interact electrically and vibrationally with its external cellular environments. Thus, a communication circuit of energetic information is established between the DNA and the cell. "It means your cells routinely use electrogenetics to control almost every activity," Horowitz points out.[34] However, when the electrical mechanisms are disrupted, cellular abnormalities follow, inhibiting proper self-regulation and regeneration processes, and ultimately, changes in the DNA result. My channels confirmed that along with the cellular response described above, my DNA had also been damaged, normal gene coding sequences had been altered, and mutations had been generated as a result of the poor quality energetic information transmitted to the DNA from the cellular membrane.

During my work with a functional medicine specialist, I agreed to undergo some genetic testing as a means of better understanding some of the root causes of my diseases. When we interpret genomic profiling results, it is important to remember that the profiles summarizing our mutations are only indicative of our propensity toward expressing a certain "phenotype," which is the formal term for a certain disease or medical condition. The information is based on the gene sequencing errors or variations in the coded portion of the chromosome that science can currently measure—in other words, the biological DNA. It is an indication of the potential we have of actually expressing a disease associated with those mutations, but it is not a guarantee. Depending on the contributing factors that influence the integrity of the energy in our personal quantum field, as described previously, and how these influence the information provided to our cells and thus our genes, by our quantum DNA, we may never manifest these diseases at all. In fact, this suggests it is likely that genetic variations (mutations) are not the root cause of disease at all. Rather it is the energetic environment that influences a person's susceptibility to environmental factors, through the energetic information provided, that creates a higher risk for disease. Accordingly, as cellular signaling and transport mechanisms become dysfunctional as a result of poor energetic conditions in our personal quantum fields, incorrect messages are transmitted to the biological DNA instruction sets to re-encode (transcribe) the genes for errant cellular responses instead. This process is known as "genetic transcription," which results in the mutations that genomic profiling results reveal. Mutations are then perpetuated as cellular division continues to copy the incorrect gene sequences, increasing the risk for disease. Unfortunately, under normal circumstances, once created, genetic mutations cannot be repaired.

It is important to note here that the genomic testing results, then, were simply evidence of the fact that the energetic integrity of my personal quantum field had been compromised so severely by the factors I described earlier, that cellular malfunction, DNA damage, as well as mutations, occurred as a result. Based on this, my compromised quantum field likely had more of an impact on the manifestation of my poor health than any influence or increased risk due to normal genetic variation and biological inheritance factors. To me, the results were not only proof of this mechanism but also an indication of how far the influence of all these factors had gone in my body.

My genomic profiling results indicated that I had some interesting genetic variations—known as single nucleotide polymorphisms, or SNPs (pronounced *snips*)—that support the energetic disease mechanisms provided. SNPs are variations in the genetic code that occur at certain places on our DNA, resulting from a substitution in individual nucleotide bases along the DNA strand during the replication process. In other words, there is a deviation from the normal base pairing sequence rules (A with T, and C with G), creating a change in information sequencing or genetic code. Some inherited genetic variation influences the differences we see in height and eye color, for example. It is generally presumed that most naturally occurring genetic variations have little or no effect on our phenotype, that is, on our physiology and our propensity for disease.[35] However, although not all SNPs affect our health, some in particular were certainly evidence of some of physiological dysfunction and disease mechanisms that had occurred in my case. This was a sobering reminder for me of just how severe my condition had become. Ordinarily, I might have felt my future prospects were quite dire and my fate sealed given this evidence, but I remained hopeful, since I now had a much better grasp of the true mechanisms of genetics and disease and what could be done to rectify my situation.

Among the myriad of mutations reported, the most notable were those that could definitively be correlated to my symptoms and diagnoses. In particular, there were SNPs that indicated a high predisposition for chronic inflammation, the mechanism by which the body repairs those cells and tissues that have been damaged. It is also the primary defense mechanism of our immune system against allergens, viruses, bacteria, and yeast, many of which I had struggled with from time to time since childhood. My results also reported the presence of multiple SNPs indicative of the presence of cytokines, which help regulate the inflammation response, as described earlier. As I discovered firsthand, when inflammation becomes excessive, it causes substantial cellular damage and numerous disease states.

My methylation genetic profile indicated the presence of mutations related to improper enzyme functioning. These enzymes affect neurotransmitter activity, which regulates everything from sleep and mood to pain sensitivity. Additional neurotransmitter testing supported these results and showed abnormal levels for some of the major ones including serotonin, dopamine, and norepinephrine. Thus, cell structural changes and the corresponding alterations in intracellular signaling molecule function (including cytokines and neurotransmitters) described earlier, may very well have been responsible for the genetic mutations seen in the results.

Mutations indicative of the propensity for mast cell (tumor cell) activation and a potential inability to repair DNA were also identified in the profiling results. The detoxification profile generated as part of the genomic testing revealed the presence of SNPs that most likely correlated with my inability to detoxify various toxins, owing to the compromise of certain cellular enzymes. This would certainly have predisposed me to cancer by the electrical cellular mechanisms described.

As indicated, coding errors and physical abnormalities in the chromosome can also be caused by toxic chemicals, radiation, and free radicals, all of which I had been exposed to. The altered cellular dysfunction that results can cause abnormal growth, malignant transformation, and perpetuation of tumor cells.

Fluctuating oxygen levels will result in fluctuations in the types of genes that are activated, among other things. . . . Hypoxia and acidic tumor microenvironments will cause certain genes to become activated and expressed, while other genes may become inactivated so that the metabolic reactions within tumor cells will be altered. These conditions can also create DNA damage and impair DNA electrochemical repair mechanisms.[36]

Research has shown that "contacts and connections with the extracellular matrix (ECM) and neighboring cells break down in cancer cells. The change in connections of the cytoskeletal proteins with the ECM components, and the cell membrane, disrupts the flow of inward current into cancer cells, [and] affects their genetic activity."[37] In many cancers, it appears that it is not a failure of the immune system that triggers cellular demise, it is the failure of the DNA repair mechanism.[38] In any case, the evidence was once again indicative of what had transpired at a physical level.

Not surprisingly, there were also many SNPs present that are correlated with inflammation-related conditions and disease. One particular gene, the ERAP1 gene on one of my chromosomes, turned out later to be a telling piece of evidence of what seemed to be at play, as this mutation is commonly associated with inflammation. This gene provides instructions for making an enzyme that normally regulates and reduces inflammation by cleaving cytokine receptor proteins and inhibiting their cellular signaling. The enzyme also functions in controlling immunity by assisting in mechanisms that trigger infected cells to self-destruct. Under mutated conditions, it was clear how both my ability to control inflammation and immunity had been compromised.[39] Many other SNPs were reported that are typically associated with cancer.

Lastly, the results indicated some potential issues associated with the cytochrome C protein complex, discussed earlier. It is possible that these had created an aversion or resistance to apoptosis, which is considered to be one of the main hallmarks of cancer and tumor formation. In contrast to apoptosis, when cells are acutely damaged under traumatic or necrotic conditions, as they were in my case, the cell explodes and releases contents into the cellular environment. This results in cytotoxic conditions that can damage surrounding tissue and harm other molecules, which I was told was part of the reason I experienced so much physical pain and discomfort.

Despite the despairingly negative and unpromising results from the genomic profiling results, I was relieved and very encouraged when I subsequently learned that it is possible, through our own consciousness, to alter the information in our personal quantum field to activate our quantum DNA. This newly activated or improved information is then transmitted by the quantum DNA to our physical DNA, initiating a DNA re-coding response for more efficient mechanisms of self-regulation, regeneration, and repair. These enhanced coding instructions are transmitted to the cells and DNA to shift them toward the cessation of cellular and genetic disease processes and abnormalities and toward healing and normal biological functioning.

> **Despite the despairingly negative and unpromising results from the genomic profiling results, I was relieved and very encouraged when I subsequently learned that it is possible, through our own consciousness, to alter the information in our personal quantum field to activate our quantum DNA.**

8

Healing through Consciousness

Expressing Purposeful and Genuine Intent to Heal

Ultimately, healing the physical form does nothing unless there is a complementary change in consciousness. All healers know this. If this does not take place, the physical form will return rather rapidly to the state it was in.

DAVID SPANGLER[1]

HEALING

Holistic healing modalities emphasize that healing involves a much deeper level of change and transformation at all levels of the individual. It is different than curing, which is defined as occurring when the signs and symptoms of a disease disappear and any medication, surgery, or other form of intervention is no longer required. As Dr. Larry Malerba points out, "Most conventional doctors do not concern themselves with the whole; they tend to consider the job done when the specific part in question is no longer generating symptoms. . . . Authentic healing is almost always accompanied by a change and growth of consciousness." In actuality, there is no finite outcome that is achieved in healing, and so it may be seen more appropriately as a continuum. It is a process of self-evolvement that is never quite complete, as there are always opportunities for growth and improvement.[2] Healing is a journey that, through the development of our conscious awareness, can lead to full recovery from disease, permanently. It may take place over many years, which may be a daunting and discouraging prospect for some. It is not always a quick fix and certainly not something that can be administered to the patient by a health practitioner in a single injection or treatment. Healing requires full and genuine participation of the individual for whom the change is desired. Disease and the challenges it presents are an opportunity for those who are ill to embrace and embody the transformation it can potentially bring. When we are openly and genuinely committed to the healing process, disease may no longer be seen as an inconvenience and an invitation to suffer. Healing allows us to move beyond the diagnosis and treatment stages of disease and look at the real underlying causes of what makes us ill to find deeper triggers and, thus, potential solutions. Doctors may remark to some with chronic or incurable diseases that "there is nothing more they can do." This kind of sentiment only teaches us that we cannot or are not supposed to get well. Wisdom teaches us that there is hope; we can improve our chances of healing when we apply ourselves genuinely and appropriately to this end.

As I continued to move forward in my new role as practitioner, it became apparent to me that many of my clients and people I know are actually afraid of healing. To them, predictable situations, as miserable as they might be, are still better than the unknown. Despite the fact that many of our emotions and thoughts have Akashic drivers, which can be altered as I have explained, and that we are not consciously aware of these aspects, some are still too frightened of what they might discover about themselves in the process. Most of the root causes of disease lie beneath the surface. Our subconscious mind or soul has gathered information that serves as the drivers for disease, without the involvement of the conscious mind; yet, we continue to feel guilty or blame ourselves for the way we are. Admittedly, I was also afraid in the beginning, but after my Akashic

Records (soul programs and contracts) were cleared, these feelings dissipated, and I felt much more confident and able to see things objectively, from a less personal and victimized standpoint. I began to appreciate that healing is a learning opportunity for the soul rather than an unwelcome event in our lives. The process can teach us things about ourselves that we might not have paid attention to otherwise. Sometimes, we have to be really uncomfortable or even desperate before we are ready to listen to the messages our bodies are giving us. That was certainly the case for me. To this day, I am grateful for the catalyst for change that disease presented to me. In many ways, it was truly a gift.

We need to remind ourselves that we can and were designed to self-heal and regulate our bodies. We can change this information and the self-limiting beliefs and perceptual patterns to effect real change in our bodies. From a quantum perspective, these aspects of ourselves are nothing more than energetic information, represented as frequencies, stored in nonlocal realms. Through our own consciousness, we can access the limitless intelligence available to us, stored holographically as information in our Akashic Records within our personal quantum field. We can utilize this information to change our DNA blueprint by applying and substituting new or different frequencies. We are far from helpless. As co-creators of our own reality, we can manifest changes and improvements in our health simply by changing the information our DNA blueprint uses as the basis for the biological DNA instruction sets that govern the body's healing mechanisms. It is about drawing on the energies of the past held in our Akashic Records to activate our quantum DNA and, in doing so, reactivate the memory of who we truly are—healthy, vital, balanced, and self-regulating biological organisms. This, in my mind, is healing. We have simply forgotten how this works.

SUCCESSFUL APPROACHES TO HEALING

While I experienced some healing as a result of energy treatments and soul work I undertook over a period of several years, changes did not occur at deeper levels involving cellular and genetic alterations. Although the vibrational energy medicine treatments helped to increase my life-force energy, raise my vibration level, and successfully treat both my jaw cancer and the synovial lesion in my hip, my overall physical health did not improve in an appreciable way. The soul work assisted in clearing the subconscious mind and soul programs from my Akashic Records resulting in a release of discordant, self-limiting, and nonproductive energies and replacement with more supportive and positive ones. This work resulted in the disappearance of both the occipital and sacral tumors, eliminating my allergies, and improving my insomnia issues, but they were only the start of the journey. Collectively, these modalities afforded me sufficient clarity, balance, and strength so that I could continue to explore the root causes of my physiological dysfunction and disease states as well as the approaches to healing that were successful in the end. I was determined to come out the other side of this experience and, if I did, share the knowledge and experience I acquired in the process with others and, above all, with my clients.

Ultimately, it was the tools that involved working with the quantum aspect of my DNA through my own consciousness that created the real change at the cellular and genetic level, and therefore, this is what I focus on in the descriptions that follow. I maintain that the reason for my success was that, in my case, healing did not occur until I activated the energies and memories held within my quantum DNA and used this information to communicate different instructions to my cells to initiate repair and regeneration activities. I expect that this is likely the case for many with chronic, deep-seated, and pervasive kinds of diseases, such as cancer, autoimmune, or genetically inherited diseases. If there is ineffective communication between our quantum and biological DNA, providing improper or insufficient information to our cells, we may simply be unable to address the underlying cause of our disease or respond to treatment of any kind. This is a critically important point.

> If there is ineffective communication between our quantum and biological DNA, providing improper or insufficient information to our cells, we may simply be unable to address the underlying cause of our disease or respond to treatment of any kind.

The tools I employed to achieve success are fundamentally different than any other forms of healing that I had been exposed to or tried in the past. The main distinction is that these involved working more extensively with energy in a quantum, multidimensional, and nonlocal way, as opposed to the three-dimensional "Earth energies" that characterize some of the more traditional forms of energy medicine. These traditional approaches typically focus on clearing blocks and re-establishing flow and energetic balance to the subtle energy bodies. Some of the more advanced forms work with more localized energy signals that when transmitted and applied, prompt the body to respond in areas and ways that are needed most. The healer poses as the delivery agent for these energies, but the patient's own consciousness as the inner healer is not always actively engaged in facilitating a change as a result of the energies that are introduced. It has been my observation that our DNA, Innate Self, and Higher Self are not necessarily directly nor intentionally involved in these processes. Allopathic approaches appear to give even less credence to the intelligence of our bodies or DNA in the process of healing.

In those modalities covered here, the patient intentionally provides permission and allows for new or different quantum information to be transmitted to activate their quantum DNA and alter the DNA blueprint via the Innate Self. The Innate Self in turn informs the cells to change the three-dimensional chemistry of the body and the genes follow suit. Thus, energetic information changes chemistry. In this simple yet very profound way, we are truly orchestrators of our own healing processes—but in order to do so successfully, we need to tell our DNA and our cells what we want to create. Nature has designed them to respond to our conscious intent and the instructions embodied in this intent. The opportunity for change resides in the fact that we are able to exercise conscious choice, through pure intent. Nothing will happen if we do not want it to happen, or if we do not instruct our Innate Self to respond differently to what is happening in our bodies. We are far less likely to be successful if we simply acquiesce to our own fate and we unconditionally accept our disease state. We must circumvent the autonomic control the brain and its logic has over the body in a conscious, concerted way in order to heal. I felt immensely empowered by this important realization.

The opportunity for change resides in the fact that we are able to exercise conscious choice, through pure intent.

There are countless stories describing patients with serious or terminal conditions who, by upholding positive beliefs about themselves and the eradication of their own disease and by consciously employing some form of intention with regards to their desire to heal, have experienced complete and seemingly miraculous recoveries.

The Institute of Noetic Sciences has gathered together all scientifically recorded cases of so-called miracle cures. Although the received wisdom is that these cases are rare, a scan of the medical literature is instructive. One in eight skin cancers heals spontaneously, as does nearly one in five genitourinary cancers. Virtually all types of illnesses including diabetes, Addison's disease, and atherosclerosis, where vital organs or body parts are supposedly irretrievably damaged, have spontaneously healed. A small body of research concerns terminal cancer patients who, with little or no medical intervention, end up beating the odds. . . . Many cases of spontaneous remission seem to occur after someone makes a massive psychological shift and re-creates a life that is engaging and purposeful.[3]

In his book *The Holographic Universe,* Michael Talbot said:

The power of conscious intention in directing our own healing processes is unbelievably potent. It is applied in exactly the same manner as practitioners would in their own healing work, by focusing on their desire to manifest a particular outcome in the treatment session. In a holographic universe, we are connected to our bodies through our consciousness. If our body is a reflection of the whole, then there must be all kinds of mechanisms to control what's going on.[4]

As Sondra Barrett also points out, "this holographic matrix provides each cell with its cellular mind. This discovery that every cell contains a reflection of the whole has given us a tremendous clue to how our mysterious, multilevel body is constructed."[5] Consciousness, therefore, is the key to healing. The strongest influence available to alter our DNA is our own consciousness. It literally changes the frequency of our DNA.

Consciousness, therefore, is the key to healing. The strongest influence available to alter our DNA is our own consciousness. It literally changes the frequency of our DNA.

Through our own consciousness, when we can access quantum holographic information contained at the nonlocal level and exchange this for erroneous information that has not served our bodies well, the possibilities for healing are astounding. "Our consciousness can talk to the cellular structure of our own body and serves to strengthen our immune system and chase away disease, because the energy of human consciousness is in actual fact, information energy. It sends instructions for our body to shift."[6]

Quantum information is readily accessible, and because it is holographic, we are not separate from it. It is not really outside of us; it is everywhere—it transcends time and space. As I have personally demonstrated, through our own consciousness, we can alter the discordant energy in our personal quantum fields to influence the state of our own health and our physical bodies. Although a person may feel more supported and empowered throughout the healing process through the work of practitioners, it is actually the self that initiates and allows the healing. It does not occur as a direct result of a practitioner's intervention on the patient's behalf without their conscious involvement and intent.

> It is actually the self that initiates and allows the healing. It does not occur as a direct result of a practitioner's intervention on the patient's behalf without their conscious involvement and intent.

OVERCOMING BARRIERS TO HEALING

In order to realize the benefits of working with our consciousness in affecting our health, it is important to appreciate that healing and transformation comes from inside (not outside) ourselves. We must work from the inside out to effect change. My circumstances clearly demonstrate the impact that emotional, mental, and spiritual factors have on how things play out for us in terms of our cellular and genetic response. As difficult as it may seem at times, these should not be viewed as impediments to progress, but as opportunities for change. We are more likely to be destined for failure if we remain stuck in our personal or societal self-limiting beliefs that tell us it is in our genes, or our disease has made us a victim of uncontrollable events for which there is no recourse. There is no need to believe that we do not deserve perfection in our own bodies. The fears we possess about ourselves and around disease are often unsubstantiated and rarely real. They are simply grounded in the dual nature and physical limitations of our three-dimensional reality with little or no regard for what is possible when we move to a much broader definition of why we truly become ill and how we can heal given our quantum nature. The approaches allopathic medicine sometimes takes might lead people to believe that if we are really sick, then we must require some kind of major intervention or treatment. Instead, the solutions can be remarkably simple when we embrace the truth that we are designed and meant to heal. Ultimately, our cells and DNA are a reflection of the divinity that resides within each and every one of us. It is usually the conscious mind and soul program energies generating beliefs, thoughts, and emotions that cloud our perceptions and prevent either our own admission or recollection of this important truth. For me, these realizations represented a major turning point in my feelings toward myself, my physiological dysfunction, and disease, as well as my attitude about future prospects for healing.

In reality, it is our own conscious empowerment over the energy that resides in our personal quantum field that is the solution to changing our DNA blueprint and re-encoding our genes. Part of the magic of working with consciousness tools is that they take us beyond the limitations of our own minds. As Barbara Ann Brennan points out:

> The holographic experience requires expanded awareness. It requires great sensitivity to what is, both personally and interpersonally. It is possible to develop this expanded awareness in a step-by-step manner. . . . This holographic experience is the experience of the healing moment. When linear time and three-dimensional space are transcended, healing automatically takes place. This is the true nature of the universe.[7]

No amount of willpower can overcome the conditions that lead to the energetic underpinnings of disease I have described. As I have alluded to, it is next to impossible to achieve permanent resolution without addressing the causal nature of who we are, particularly at the soul level. Healing has to take place at all levels of our being, the emotional, mental, and spiritual levels in addition to the physical. It is an integrative process in which the body-mind-spirit cannot be separate. We cannot just decide to be different. We need to surrender to ourselves and to the healing process, unconditionally and in the absence of ego. Two of the biggest reasons that people do not heal is that they are afraid and cannot let go. As some say, "resistance is persistence." This was most certainly true in my case, and I found that the real work began when I finally surrendered and truly embodied a genuine intent to heal. It is most often more important to *allow* than to understand the precise mechanism for our disease. When we focus mentally and emotionally on the disease itself, we tend to bring our attention to the physical body itself and the superficial causes of disease described by medical science, often to the degree that it becomes a part of our identity. We need to release tightly held aspects of ourselves that only serve to perpetuate the condition and our often desperate need to control the situation in times of illness. Furthermore, it isn't even necessary to have a firm medical diagnosis or to know what is happening to us at a genetic or a cellular level, as I have explained here, in order to heal.

We do not need to understand the inner workings of the universe or details of quantum energies, nor do we need to be spiritually gifted or profoundly intuitive, to accomplish profound results in healing. We only need to work with our consciousness, Higher Self, and Innate Self in ways that are described in the next chapter to achieve success. None of the approaches requires a specific religious or spiritual belief system, only an ability to work consciously with the context of our quantum multidimensionality.

> **"**
> We do not need to understand the inner workings of the universe or details of quantum energies, nor do we need to be spiritually gifted or profoundly intuitive, to accomplish profound results in healing. **"**

INTENTION AS A VEHICLE FOR CONSCIOUSNESS

In the various practices and techniques that I have either been exposed to or have employed myself, using one's consciousness to manifest any kind of result involves working with intention. Working with intention is the method by which we set the energy in motion to solicit a response or outcome from our desires or wishes on behalf of our consciousness. Establishing an intention is much like stating the purpose or objective of a particular request. It establishes the scope of work for that request.

An intention assists us in demonstrating our sincerity and the genuineness of our desire to achieve a positive outcome that is for our greater good. Because everything is vibration, even intention is a frequency. At a basic level, it creates a positive frequency within one's personal quantum field to augment the energetic shifts we are making. Expressing our intent and asking our Innate Self and Higher Self for the help we need to heal is also critically important. This is because the prevailing laws of the universe and mankind are predicated on the concept of free will. Nothing will happen unless we exercise choice and give ourselves, our cells, and our DNA permission. Although many aspects of our lives are predetermined through our divine plan and what we as souls have expressed as our desire for learning prior to our incarnation, we have a choice as to how we respond to the experiences we face and how we govern ourselves.

> We are who we are by design, not by accident. Every detail is our soul's choice: how and where we live; our strengths, talents, and abilities; our family of origin and the circumstances of our birth; our career path; our friends, lovers, children. These details are ideal for us at this time. The life we find ourselves leading, the personality we sport, the body we inhabit, every particular of our existence is organized to support us in coming to know our soul's perfection, to know our Divine essence no matter what our conditions or circumstances.[8]

We cannot blame fate, much less our genes, for our health when we have choices. Through the consciousness tools described next, and possibly others that may be similar, we are expressing our choices through our intention. We can consciously choose to access the energies associated with the qualities and attributes we desire to help us with personal growth, healing, and manifesting all that is for our best and highest good. We must consciously express our intent to heal, to change, or transform; otherwise, we remain stuck in our dysfunctional ways and in ill health.

I first began working with conscious intention when I learned to do Shamanic journeys some time ago, and it is now standard protocol for the channeling and healing work that I currently do. This same approach is used here in the consciousness and DNA exercises. Intention is what allows us to connect our three-dimensional physical reality with quantum, multi-dimensional fields of information through our consciousness. It creates a gateway or a portal that allows us access to the energy that resides there in a dedicated and focused way. Because we are using our conscious intent to access something that is quantum, however, the response we receive via our consciousness may not be recognizable in a linear sort of way or manifest as we might expect. When we heal, sometimes it is necessary to surrender our need to understand or to know why things are happening as they are.

Intentions should come from a heart-centered place, in the absence of ego or self-judgment, accompanied by a real desire to receive the help, information, or change we are asking for. They should be concise and presented during any exercise with focus and a sense of presence. The objectives established as part of our intention should be clear or the response or reaction we receive may likewise be unclear. We also need to be cognizant of any tendencies we may have to establish multiple agendas or contingencies to our plan. We need to understand our purpose and why we have chosen that particular purpose, as well as establish some basic parameters for the response we are expecting (without establishing full conscious control of the outcome). Throughout our consciousness exercises, we should also try to keep our intention mindful, active, and in a state of present-moment awareness.

Intention is not a new concept and has been employed successfully in the past to achieve proven results in many of these applications, under controlled experimental laboratory conditions. There is a large body of research regarding the effects of intention on altering physical matter, influencing events, and in healing. A good deal of this is well summarized in Lynne McTaggart's book *The Intention Experiment*. McTaggart cites specific experiments conducted by scientists Ghosh and Zeilinger as being the key to a science of intention and how thoughts are able to affect finished, solid matter.

> They suggest that the observer effect occurs not simply in the world of the quantum particle, but also in the world of the everyday. Things no longer should be seen to exist in and of themselves, but like a quantum particle, exist only in relationship. Co-creation and influence may be a basic, inherent property of life. Our observation of every component in our world may help to determine its final state . . . the physical world and matter itself appears to be malleable, susceptible to influence from the outside.[9]

Experiments have been conducted to examine the effect of energy sent by healers and meditators through established intentions. Findings revealed that when someone holds a focused thought, it may actually be altering the molecular structure of the object of their intention.[10] Researchers Gary Schwartz and Melinda Connor studied master healers when they were "running energy" by using their intentions and concluded that directed intention appears to manifest itself as both electrical and magnetic energy that can be measured. This lent itself strongly to the supposition that intention generates frequencies that are capable of mediating healing. Subsequent studies of biophoton emissions by Schwartz revealed that healing intention creates light and what he believed were some of the most organized (coherent) light waves found in nature.[11] The notion of the creation of coherent frequencies is fundamental to our understanding of how conscious intention could have such far-reaching effects on physical aspects of our body and our cells. Intention may be capable of focusing energy on our DNA and cells to create coherent signals and an appropriately orchestrated healing response. German biophysicist Herbert Frölich developed a model that showed

> living energy is able to organize to one giant coherent state, with the highest form of quantum order known to nature. When subatomic particles are said to be "coherent" or "ordered," they become highly interlinked by bands of common electromagnetic fields and resonate like a multitude of tuning forks all attuned to the same frequency. They stop behaving like anarchic individuals and begin operating like one well-rehearsed marching band.[12]

McTaggart cites numerous sources describing the effect that vivid visualization techniques, which are a form of conscious intention, have on treating illness. She indicates that

> patients have boosted treatment of an array of acute and chronic conditions from coronary artery disease and high blood pressure to low-back pain and musculoskeletal diseases, including fibromyalgia, by using mental pictures and metaphoric representations of their bodies fighting the illness. Visualization has also improved postsurgical outcomes, helped with pain management, and minimized the side effects of chemotherapy.[13]

Biofeedback and autogenic relaxation techniques also demonstrate our ability to consciously control many of our body's functions such as blood pressure, body temperature, heart rate, and breathing as well as many of the symptoms associated with disease.

As McTaggart points out, working with intention is not a special gift but a learned skill that is readily taught and can be used in many aspects of our daily lives.[14] Exercises are included in her book that are designed to help individuals become more effective in using intention. These have been extrapolated from the success that was achieved in the laboratory experiments she documents and has participated in. McTaggart provides guidance on setting up intention space, calibrating conscious awareness, maintaining attention and focus, stating intentions and specificity, as well as tips on visualization and getting ourselves out of the way. This may be particularly helpful for those who have no previous background or exposure to meditation, yoga, and spiritual activities such as channeling, journeying, or other forms of connecting on a deeper level with ourselves and nonordinary forms of reality.

THE EXPERIENCE OF CONSCIOUS INTENTION

The experience of consciousness is unique and deeply personal. As a result, there are a multitude of ways of experiencing it. In other words, reality, as seen through the eye of the beholder, is different for each and every person. We each experience it through our own individual perceptual filters and the lens of "you"—one's own beliefs; imagination; sensory sensitivities to visual, auditory, and sentient cues; and who we are at every level. There is no right or wrong way to experience consciousness. It is what we create, and it transpires in our own field of awareness. In response to the intentions we express, images (like a movie clip) may appear in what is often referred to as our mind's eye, or inner sight. We might visualize the action of our intention by observing ourselves as if watching it with another pair of eyes. We might see our own body (or a part of our body), our cells or DNA, or even some kind of tangible energy as the subject of the images that are projected. We might hear the sound of our own voice, the voice of our Higher Self, or some other unrecognizable voice who speaks as the voice of our intention, as though it were providing the inaudible, mental instructions to our Higher Self and Innate Self that we wish to implement. Some evidence suggests that mental instructions may be more important than any actual visual image we might conjure in our conscious awareness.[15] But, it is a personal choice, and what works for some may not work for others. Some might be able to feel energy as waves or vibrations or perhaps notice a different feeling in their physical or energetic bodies. Others may not be able to see, hear, or feel anything, yet they may have an overwhelming sense of knowing what is occurring as a result of their intention. A subtle shift or change, an outcome, or some indication of the success of one's intention might be sensed in some way. Even if nothing is apparent at any level of conscious awareness, it does not mean that nothing is happening. In true quantum fashion, the outcome of our intentions is the ultimate proof of their power and influence. The biggest challenge for those who are beginning to work with conscious intention usually is in trusting in the *realness* of this nonphysical experience, despite its perceived intangibility, and whatever response or outcome that it may generate.

Some may attribute a vague, almost ethereal quality to their experiences of consciousness. This is to be expected since we are experiencing a shift in our three-dimensional perception during these exercises to a much different, nonlinear, and quantum state of reality. Things will rarely appear as our logically trained mind wants them to appear. Rather, what is revealed to us is usually the message or metaphor that Spirit or our Higher Self wants to appear, providing wisdom, guidance, or understanding about our intention or healing processes. As we continue to work with these exercises and expand our conscious awareness, we may find that we are able to experience these events with increasing mental acuity and detail.

> **"**
> The biggest challenge for those who are beginning to work with conscious intention usually is in trusting in the *realness* of this nonphysical experience, despite its perceived intangibility, and whatever response or outcome that it may generate. **"**

During my own consciousness exercises and personal practice, there is almost always a reduced sense of my physical self, akin to a loss in the awareness of the boundary of my physical body beyond the feeling of my body mass and skin. Perhaps in some way this is indicative of my ability to sense my subtle energetic bodies as opposed to the way we would typically experience the physical body, as dense matter or a solid substance. This sets the stage (metaphorically and realistically) for what transpired in my exercises in terms of the connection or merging of my own consciousness with my personal quantum field. During these sessions, I remain cognizant and aware of my external surroundings; I am still relaxed and calm. Although there is a perceptible shift during these exercises, I would not describe them as completely altered states of consciousness or out-of-body experiences. They are most often accompanied by a very recognizable sense of love and compassion and are reassuringly pleasant, positive states of awareness, as one might expect.

Many people have specific or sacred spaces where activities such as meditation or personal practices and rituals are carried out. I typically carry out these sessions at relatively the same time and in the same location in my home. I usually conduct them lying down or sitting comfortably in a space that is dedicated to my spiritual practice and writing, in the early morning before the day becomes full of demands and mental distractions. This serves to promote relaxation, create a sense of familiarity, and facilitate commitment and dedication to the session. There is also evidence that other quantum effects are generated as a result. Experiments suggests that

> the constant replaying of ordered thoughts seemed to be changing the physical reality of the room, and making the quantum virtual particles of empty space more "ordered." And then, like a domino effect, the "order" of the space appeared to assist the outcome of the experiment. . . . Carrying out the intentions in one particular space appeared to enhance their effects over time.[16]

In other words, the ordering process of intention appears to carry on, perpetuating and possibly even intensifying its charge. Obviously, this can create an incredibly powerful effect.

Working effectively with conscious intention in these circumstances requires us to release any semblance of conscious control or ego. This is absolutely critical, in my opinion, to achieving success. Instead of completely self-directing our affairs down to the minutiae, we have to trust that our Innate Self and Higher Self are in charge, and whatever transpires is for our best and highest good. If we are clear and specific with our intentions, we can assume that the message and its meaning is understood and will be executed appropriately.

Finally, we must surrender to the process underway and be able to let go of our understanding of what is happening. It is normal to want to control things—even I did in the beginning, but I found that my ability to let go improved dramatically with time. We need to release our attachment to any outcome for the session, other than the expectations we hold for healing as a result of the intention we have expressed.

9

Consciousness Tools
for Healing

Working with Quantum Tools
That Heal and Transform

Whatever else it may contain, the Akashic experience conveys the sense that the experiencing subject is not separate from the objects of his or her experience—the sense that "I, the experiencing subject, am linked in subtle but real ways to other people and to nature." In deeper experiences of this kind there is a sense that "the cosmos and I are one."

In its many variations . . . it comes from somewhere beyond our brain and body and . . . the information on which it is based is conserved somewhere beyond our brain and body. The Akashic experience gives clear testimony that we are connected to an information and memory field objectively present in nature.

ERVIN LASZLO[1]

TRANSFORMATIONAL SOUND AND
BREATH EXERCISES

After the radiation therapy I received for my spinal tumor, my physical condition began to deteriorate. There had been no improvement in my musculoskeletal issues, and I was in a lot of pain, particularly in my back and hips. I was exhausted, stiff, and sore. Walking any appreciable distance was difficult. I saw a spiritual medium who noted that my breathing was poor and recommended the technique developed by Judith Kravitz called Transformational Breath. In a guided meditation format, the technique utilizes a high vibrational energy force created by a specific breathing pattern, combined with the power of vocal sounds to promote healing on all levels: mental, emotional, spiritual, and physical.

The primary objective of the Transformational Breath technique is to open up the respiratory system; this alleviates restricted breathing patterns that are created unconsciously, often to suppress unpleasant or undesirable memories and feelings. The source of these imprinted patterns originates in the subconscious mind and soul's records, as I described in earlier chapters. At the beginning of a Transformational Breath session, participants have the option of invoking the guidance and assistance of spiritual guides and entities (which the individual may or may not be aware of) in creating a sacred experience in which the possibility to co-create and manifest results is greatly enhanced. There is an opportunity to establish an intention that focuses the participants' conscious awareness on the desired energy and self-attributes that they would like to create.

Participants are then guided to breathe into any protected or restricted areas that can be sensed in the body in order to bring awareness and energy into those parts. This releases the blocked energy that is held there, enhancing the flow of energy and allowing for the reintegration of the energy into more harmonious, coherent patterns. At specified intervals during the exercise, participants are encouraged to use vocalized sound (*toning*) as a means of releasing and moving the energy to create more openness in the breath and in their feelings. The sound introduces higher frequencies of energy that serve to enhance and reinforce the higher vibration level being generated by the breathing.

Guided portions of the exercise assist by providing positive self-affirmations and statements that encourage participants to release and reprogram the limiting beliefs and perceptions that are created by these subconscious mind and soul programs. The Transformational Breath technique reportedly allows individuals to access the deepest and purest aspects of themselves—the spiritual self—unconditionally and without judgment during these higher vibrational states of awareness. In this way, issues are addressed at the root, or causal, level so that they are permanently resolved. In some cases, it is said that spontaneous healing results.

I followed the established exercise on a regular basis for over a year. After that, I began to use the framework of the breathing pattern and toning as the basis to create a more unique, individualized approach. I worked extensively with establishing various conscious intentions for these exercises, focusing first on releasing undesirable emotions and thoughts that I had become aware of over the course of my healing journey. Sometimes I was able to identify prevailing emotions such as fear; anger; low self-esteem and sense of self-worth; impatience; and judgment. Other times, I was unable to label them, particularly if they emanated from a deeper source in the subconscious mind or at the soul level. It did not matter, as the point was in expressing my intent to release them, no matter what they were. From there, I began to establish intentions more specifically related to manifesting changes at the cellular level, including those that would address my issues with inflammation, cellular functioning, and physical compromise. Eventually, I began to include some of the techniques described below such as communicating with my cells and substituting frequencies in my Akash to alter my DNA.

As I began to learn more about sound healing, I varied the toning portion of the exercise, substituting vowel sounds that are typically associated in sound healing with each of the energy chakras, as well as extending the length of time dedicated to generating sounds. Sometimes, I would focus my intention and direct the sound toward certain chakras and the corresponding areas of the body in which I was experiencing difficulty, such as the hip (sacral chakra), the jaw tumor (throat chakra), or the breast cancer (heart chakra) areas. The variations came quite intuitively, and I would make sounds that I could feel resonate in my body in the desired location or that felt good, sometimes vocalizing the sound, other times humming to create deeper vibration within my body. Each vertebra in the spine has a different resonant frequency, and I experimented with sounds that created reverberations in areas of my skeletal structure that were particularly problematic and where I had experienced injury, trauma, and pain. I also researched the resonant frequency of certain disease states and medical conditions to establish certain healing tones that I incorporated into the exercise using sound-generating software that I had acquired.

By this time, my own spiritual gifts and abilities were beginning to surface. I began to take on clients and conduct workshops using my own unique versions of this technique as a means of facilitating the clearing of energetic blocks, elevating vibration levels, and controlling pain in others. In the majority of cases, participants exhibited extremely positive responses on all levels as a result of these exercises. Most reported experiencing higher energy levels and states of conscious awareness, enhanced mental and emotional clarity, as well as less pain and discomfort.

Conscious Breathing

Breathing techniques have been around in ancient mind-body-spirit practices for thousands of years and are most commonly known in various yoga modalities. Given my favorable response, I was keen to learn about what was actually happening to my physical and energetic bodies as a result of these sessions. I stumbled upon a book written Dr. Dharma Singh Khalsa, an anesthetist and pain management specialist with a deep personal interest and devotion to the practice of kundalini yoga and meditation. His book *Meditation as Medicine* describes the neurophysiological response of the body to kundalini yoga and specifically to the main aspects that make up its foundation: breath, posture and movement, mantra (sacred vocal sounds), and mental focus. He says that most people do not breathe well enough to sustain normal health and the consequences of oxygen deprivation can create a variety of cardiovascular problems, mood disorders, pain, and immune deficiency, as well as liver and digestive issues.

It is not surprising then, that conscious breathing techniques I was using made me feel better physically, given my issues with oxidative stress and the problems it had created. Shallow breathing, which is common for many who experience pain, decreases oxygen exchange and activates our sympathetic nervous system's fight-or-flight mechanism. When this is in overdrive, our adrenal glands produce stress hormones and our musculoskeletal system goes into a taut state of preparedness. I remember attending a course on relaxation, and of course, I was as stiff as a board. I simply could not relax my muscles no matter how hard I tried.

Opiates that I was taking for pain control are also known to cause respiratory depression in response to low blood oxygen levels. More adrenaline is produced as oxygen levels decline, which then creates more anxiety and the cycle continues. This is a very common experience for those in chronic pain, just as it was for me. Laboratory test results were certainly evidence of this stress and showed my hormone levels and neurotransmitters were way out of balance. Tests also showed that I had excess levels of carbon dioxide in my blood, a condition known as "hypocapnia," which is indicative of breathing abnormalities. Breathing stimulates blood circulation, which is one of the primary mechanisms for cellular waste disposal. It is said that up to 70 percent of the toxins in the body are eliminated through our breathing; so, given my own issues of toxicity, this technique proved very beneficial for me.

Conscious breathing also tones the nervous system and impacts a part of the brain that is responsible for moderating pain. Deep, controlled rhythmic breathing shifts the body away from the sympathetic nervous system's fight-or-flight mode, allowing our parasympathetic nervous system to reprogram the sympathetic nervous system. The sympathetic nervous system is the body's primary neurological defense against disease. Thus, through intentional breathing, automatic functions become conscious ones.[2] In this way, we direct the body to cooperate with its own natural functioning mechanisms through the breath.

More importantly from an energetic perspective, we are not just bringing in oxygen when we breathe, we are bringing in life-force energy, or *prana,* which serves to maintain and increase our vibrational energy levels. Via the breathing process, "the vibration of human breath interlocks the finite magnetic field of humankind with the infinite magnetic field of the universe. The ebb and flow of breath is seen as a link to the motions and tides of the entire cosmos, outside our bodies, and within our bodies."[3] Based on the fact that quantum information is communicated to us via the electromagnetic energies that surround us, we can begin to see the importance of breath as a vehicle for this energy. Essentially, through breath work, we are able to synchronize or resonate our personal quantum fields with the universal field through vibration. The vibrational resonance and increase in life-force energy created through breathing facilitates healing by magnifying the coherence in our field and, thus, the information that can be communicated to our cells by our quantum DNA. As previously stated, the higher our vibration is, the more DNA becomes activated as we begin to have access to more quantum information. In turn, the efficiency with which our quantum and biological DNA communicate increases. We are able to draw in healing energies with our own breath as our electromagnetic field strengthens and harmonizes in this process. When we add in two additional components to breathing—sound and conscious awareness—we further enhance this effect.

> The vibrational resonance and increase in life-force energy created through breathing facilitates healing by magnifying the coherence in our field and, thus, the information that can be communicated to our cells by our quantum DNA.

Sound

The experience of sound is at the very core of human consciousness, and when coupled with positive intention, it becomes an extremely powerful tool for healing. Sound healing is founded on the premise that all matter, including every cell, organ, organ system, tissue, or bone in our physical bodies vibrates at very specific frequencies. Collectively, their vibrations work together to create a compilation of frequencies that are all in harmony with each other. The body is represented by a virtual symphony of tones, pitches, and rhythms within its midst. There may be either a propensity toward, or the presence of, disease when we exhibit a discordant or noncoherent energetic state. Various parts of the body (including our cells) may be resonating at a different frequency than is their ideal—their harmonics may be aberrant or there may be too much noise or interfering vibration for them to vibrate in tune and harmony. In some places of the body, in areas of stagnant energy, there may be no frequency at all; in others with excess energy, distorted frequencies may result. This was most certainly true in my case, and there were very definite anomalies, blocks, and irregular patterns seen by my practitioners in my energy field, corresponding to my various problems: the jaw and breast cancers, the hip dysfunction, the tumors, and areas of inflammation. Because cells function as electrical dipoles (transducers), they can convert acoustic waves to electrical waves (and vice versa)—we can see how introducing sound to the body can create positive effects by creating optimal electrical conditions that promote better DNA communication and proper cell function as discussed previously.

The sound and breath technique assisted in the transformation of the energy in my personal quantum field to a more harmonious state and an increase in its overall vibration level through a process known as "sonic entrainment." This occurs when the higher vibrational effects produced from the toning and breathing allow the body's energy to resonate or vibrate in such a way that the body's absorption frequencies match the higher frequencies being introduced. The lower vibrational energies in the body are subsequently altered as their resonant frequency shifts to that of the higher energy. In addition, if the vibration introduced by the toning is strong enough, it will overcome and entrain a weaker vibration in the body into the same stronger vibration, through a process known as "resonant dominance." In reality, however, the elevation in vibration that occurs does not necessarily mean that the body or its parts now resonate at a higher frequency per se; it means that there is a more consistent vibration with fewer distortions and distractions, in other words, more harmony and flow.[4] Every part of the body can be affected by this process, including the cells and DNA molecules, which absorb frequencies that are characteristic of their structure. When you target the resonant frequency of something, it releases energy, which the body uses naturally for the healing process.

The voice, as sound, is the ultimate healer and something our bodies and the Innate Self recognize as being inextricably linked to us.

When we create harmonics of sound, it reminds your body of something. It reminds your body of light, of deep cosmic love, and of other worlds . . . these harmonics can be utilized in incredible ways, for harmonics can evolve many things. . . . The harmonics alter something: they open the door. Certain combinations of sounds played through the human body unlock information and frequencies of intelligence.[5]

Because DNA is the same structure as our language, decoding of the information is not required. It responds to our voice by us simply talking to it. When the voice is used as an intentional healing form as I describe in my case, it is possible to therapeutically focus the voice to manifest change in our cells and DNA—whatever level of the body we choose to focus on with our intention. The toning sounds do not have to be perfect or on key because the body is responding to the harmonics created by the fundamental frequency, not the actual frequency of the vocalized sound. Harmonics are multiple tones, or "sounds within sounds," and are what give the voice its timbre and tonal colors, as well as concentrating and activating the vibrational energy of the sound.[6] The basis of toning is the vocalization of elongated tones and sustained sounds, primarily through the use of vowels (*A, E, I, O, U*). The vowels typically used in sound healing are those that correspond to each of the chakras. These are "uh" (first chakra), "oo" (second chakra), "oh" (third chakra), "ah" (fourth chakra), "ay" (fifth chakra), and "ee" (sixth and seventh chakras).

I also used a variety of other sounds, many of which I explored intuitively and creatively, depending on my intention, the area of focus in my body, or how I was feeling. Some sounds used derived from sacred origins or meanings, including *om,* or those used in mantras, chanting, and sacred songs.

Attaining the perfect frequency in toning is not nearly as important as the vibrational coherence it creates. Even if the frequency is not exact, it is possible to elicit a positive response from the consistency of sound, particularly when the positive frequency of an intention is added to this. My approach as a result of this was to ensure that I included both high, medium, and low notes in my toning voice range. Humming is an alternative to toning as the sounds are projected inward instead of outwards, producing an altogether different effect in the body.

Effects of Sound and Breath Work

Better vibrational coherence can manifest itself in us at all levels. On a physical level, as mentioned, each part of the body resonates at the frequency that it is meant to for perfect functioning and balance. This coherence restores harmony and homeostasis to the body. Here, vibratory waves have the most pronounced effect upon two of our most sensitive systems: the neurological and the endocrine. They strongly vibrate the brain and can charge the cortex of the brain—teach and entrain the brain to restore and replace weak, dormant, or missing frequencies. This can create new neural synaptic connections and improve the flow and pulse of cerebral spinal fluid. Sound affects the pituitary and hypothalamus glands, which are located through the roof of the mouth when we make toning sounds, improving glandular function. Researchers have determined techniques such as toning can also help lower heart rate and blood pressure, reduce stress hormones, enhance the release of melatonin and endorphins, improve digestion (through the stimulation of the vagus nerve), relax tension, reduce pain, and increase immune system functioning.[7]

In these ways, this technique proved to be supportive of my body throughout the healing process. As a result, I found I was far less reliant on prescription medications and treatments to moderate and lessen my symptoms. In fact, I believe I actually had fewer symptoms overall and far less fatigue than would be typical of diseases of this nature. It felt good to honor myself and know that I was able to impact my own healing process by conducting these exercises on a regular basis without the help of a practitioner. It was very empowering.

Toning and humming vibrates the body right down to the cellular level, helping our cells resonate together and release energy to stimulate activity and promote optimal cell functioning. Increased vibration actually agitates the receptor sites on the cells so that light (described earlier in our discussion of quantum information transfer) can only land on the cell's surface where the vibration is sufficient. In addition, when the vibration is higher, the propulsion of the waves through sounding structures of the body—including our cellular matrices—allows for the transmission of more light, which means more quantum information is communicated; in turn, the biological DNA becomes more efficient at relaying better instructions to the cells. I believe that increasing cellular vibration through toning and humming had the most significant effect on the positive changes I experienced at a cellular level; this in turn had the resulting effect of the ultimate change to my genetic coding. The change in charge on the surface of the cell membrane (from negative to positive), which promoted appropriate cell transport and signaling functions, was attributed largely to my work with sound. The increase in energy production at the cellular level, as well as a strengthening in the cell structure itself, were also a result of the increase in vibration produced by sound.

Interestingly, there are four core frequencies that make up the "music" in the physical DNA, each corresponding to the four nucleotide bases. A specific tone or harmonic structure is generated with certain configurations created by the precise location of the nucleotide on a particular section of the first of the double-stranded DNA—in other words, by their gene coding sequences. The second strand of DNA has the opposite sequence of frequencies so there are musical intervals at play, imparting very particular frequency characteristics to them.[8] It is likely that in the case of a mutated gene, where incorrect nucleotides are positioned on the DNA, as in sequencing errors or in the case of physically damaged DNA, a state of dissonance or disharmony may have been created. I am surmising on this basis that the effects of toning were likely to have been quite influential in affecting gene repair and re-coding.

Dr. Deepak Chopra says in his book *Quantum Healing* that the language with which we speak to our own DNA consists of primordial sounds. Chopra believes that disease occurs when there is a communication breakdown between the body, mind, and DNA. By putting primordial sound back into the body, it reminds it "what station it should be tuned to," in other words, what optimal frequency our DNA should resonate with. Chopra maintains that "starting with DNA, the whole body unfolds into many levels, and at each one . . . the sequence of sound comes first."[9]

We know from the work of Hans Jenny, who pioneered work in the field of cymatics, that it is possible to observe the effects of sound on physical matter and its ability to alter physical shape, patterns, and structure. Specific harmonics and frequencies influence water by forming larger sacred geometric forms called "structured or clustered water." It has been said that "these energetically gathered and directed forms of water are essential for optimal DNA function in the realm of electrogenetics" and that these specifically shaped clustered water molecules form the supportive (and electrically active) matrix of healthy DNA. Clustered water molecules vibrate at specific resonant frequencies, which can help restore homeostasis to the cell structures in the body.[10]

Our thoughts and feelings also consist of sound vibrations—subtle energy vibrations that vibrate at faster and higher frequencies than in our physical bodies. As aforementioned, on a mental and emotional level, sound can also reduce energy blockages and patterns due to stuck emotions, clear past traumas and memories, enhance mental capabilities, as well as accentuate positive thoughts and emotions. I found I was able to use the sound vibrations produced by toning, accompanied by positive intentions, to trigger higher energy emotions such as gratitude, compassion, love, and joy and to allow them to resonate throughout my body. Technically, these emotions are not actually higher in frequency than lower emotions of fear and anxiety, they are just more coherent and consistent tones. These emotions (as sound) stay on the same note and have no random distortion or noise, so they are characteristically more pure.

The sound and breath work undoubtedly exerted tremendous effects on my energetic state, beyond clearing my field and raising my vibration. Each of the primary energy centers of the body known as *chakras* has its own resonant frequency. Sound helps to tone and balance the energy and sculpt the energy patterns in the chakras. Discordant energies associated with thoughts, emotions, conscious mind, and soul programs will create alterations and dysfunction in the chakras. They become misshaped and deviate from their normal resonant frequency, which is typically observed by healers as a change in color (frequency). I once demonstrated the technique to one of my practitioners who monitored my energy meridians as well as my subtle energy body through her inner sight for the duration of the session. During the toning portion of the exercise, she witnessed a very strong explosion of light energy emanating outwards from my solar chakra (likely indicating the clearing of a blockage). Chakras function much like transformers, relaying external quantum information in to the internal energy field and physical body and vice versa. The flow of this information is enhanced when blockages are cleared and the chakras regain their resonant frequency. An increase in vibration was also noted by an improved quality and quantity of energy flow through each of my twelve energy meridians. My channels also indicated that this technique had a significant impact on improving my electrical flow and increasing the strength of my electromagnetic field. As discussed, these changes would have enhanced the transmission and receipt of quantum information, by the mechanisms described earlier. Based on this, I now routinely encourage my clients to utilize this technique as a powerful self-healing tool.

It is well known that working with sounds such as the binaural beat or other targeted frequencies, like those that induce theta or delta waves for example, can assist us in achieving higher states of conscious awareness. When our own vibration is raised sufficiently, it can be used to entrain us into harmony and a direct connection to our soul. There is one fundamental tone that is at the root of the existence of each one of us—a tone that represents the pure essence of who we are individually—commonly referred to as our "soul frequency." This tone is representative of our unique energetic signature and our soul. When we tone at this fundamental frequency, we essentially come home to ourselves, signaling to our bodies, cells, and DNA that this is the norm, guiding them back to home base and this vibrational point of reference. In this way, we open ourselves up through our Higher Self to unfathomable healing powers and levels of consciousness that facilitate remarkable growth, change, and transformation in us. Communication with spiritual energies and dimensions of consciousness in the nonordinary realms are also greatly enhanced when our vibration is increased.

> When we make a sound, we are connecting the solar system that we are a part of, the atomic structure and quantum mechanics that we are made of and the frequencies of our spine and auras . . . through harmonics we are connecting to all other levels that share this same mathematical structure . . . every sound we make is resonating and affecting all these other levels. . . . In particular, when we make a sound (even while simply speaking), we are resonating the mathematical structure of sound at the quantum level where we are all connected by entanglement.[11]

Sound brings the infinite to the finite through coherence and harmony, yielding an incredibly powerful outcome. I am certain that establishing a connection and resonating with higher frequencies associated with quantum fields of information through the sound and breath work, to achieve a higher vibrational energy state, contributed greatly to the success I ultimately achieved in activating my DNA and re-encoding my genes.

Sound brings the infinite to the finite through coherence and harmony, yielding an incredibly powerful outcome.

DNA MARKER ADJUSTMENT AND
PATTERN REMOVAL

As indicated in a previous chapter, there were five DNA markers illuminated in my body, each corresponding to frequency anomalies associated with the dysfunctional energetic patterns present in my personal quantum field. DNA markers are the beacons that allow us to draw in and anchor energetic soul patterns (light codes) in our physical form and are comprised of unique and complex arrays of frequencies—sets and subsets within themselves. They are within our capability to modify with our consciousness. Thus, I was able to facilitate the desired change in these markers by asking Spirit and Higher Self to call up a holographic projection of myself showing the DNA markers. With these now visible with my inner sight, I could see the color (frequency) of each one of these. Through conscious intent, I would focus on each one of the markers in turn, visualizing the correct color (frequency), while holding the desire for this correction to take place, for several minutes at a time. On one particular occasion, while performing these exercises, my channels revealed the DNA spiral, which began to unfurl as the alternate frequencies were applied. The colors began to change on the nucleotide bases that connect the two strands of the double helix. This demonstrated that the frequencies of DNA were indeed being altered in this way to change the gene coding sequences. After conducting this exercise over a period of several weeks, eventually the markers resumed their correct frequencies permanently. This is not surprising given that the power of visualization in manifesting change is demonstrated through its use in many psychological, spiritual, and energetic healing modalities. However, I felt exhilarated all the same, as the change in frequencies was evidence of the success I had achieved in working with conscious intention. I was witnessing an alteration in my own energetic patterns, without the assistance of a practitioner.

During a Quantum Healing and Hypnosis Therapy (QHHT) session that followed this work, the discordant energy patterns in my personal quantum field associated with each of the five recently altered DNA markers were removed. Even though I was under hypnosis, I was able to consciously remember the session, likely owing to my own level of spiritual awakening. Whether what was revealed during this session was a metaphor or not, I witnessed five Spiritual entities, each responsible for a specific grouping of frequencies, who removed the patterns, corrected them, and commuted them back to the universe. The relief I experienced in the aftermath of this session was immense, particularly since these patterns had been an integral part of who I was for such a long time. Now I was free of them and anxiously anticipated the healing that would come from these tremendous changes. This cemented my resolve to continue my healing journey.

As Lynne McTaggart points out, hypnosis is a type of intention in which instructions are given to our brains during an altered state. She says that hypnosis demonstrates that the brain or body is susceptible to the power of directed thought.[12] This is accomplished through communication of the brain with a portion of our consciousness that is well beyond the level of the conscious mind. The subconscious has the ability to identify all sorts of physical problems it detects within the body and, quite frequently, through hypnosis can explain the causes for the presence of illness and disease as well as its root causes. As the founder of QHHT, Dolores Cannon explains, "Very often, simply understanding why a disease is present or why a particular emotion is being experienced is sufficient for it to be relieved and removed."[13] When this is communicated to our brains, extremely profound physical and mental healing can result.

Although the energies were transmuted, I was informed that the behavioral habits would remain so that I could explore and learn from them as part of my self-work. I did as was instructed, and each day I would ask for one of the patterns to be applied to my field so that I could learn about its qualities, attributes, and their effects on me. I was no longer afraid given my newfound understanding of the soul's journey through life and the fact that my own healing had progressed to the point where many of the "aspects of self" that had created problems for me were now permanently cleared. Through this process, my perspective on life and myself has truly changed. To try these on again as though I was applying a homeopathic substance to my energy field provided a wonderful opportunity for me to appreciate how these disturbances had been created through my own negative thoughts, emotions, and limiting beliefs. I was astonished when I recognized feelings, familiar thought patterns, statements, and even some of the exact same feelings of pain and discomfort and symptoms associated with my disease. Luckily, I was able to experience them in a very neutral and detached way, observe them at a distance, and then release them from my field. As was true in my case, this is a very powerful means of transforming our DNA to promote healing, and I have worked with these particular Spiritual entities to remove these DNA markers and clear these patterns in my clients since, with the same remarkable results.

Once again, modifications to these frequencies is a quantum and multidimensional exercise, taking place outside the confines of our linear, three-dimensional reality and comprehension. When we work with our Higher Self, Innate Self, Spirit, and our consciousness, however, these activities do not necessarily have to be complicated from our point of view, as I have shown here. We connect and relate to multidimensional fields through our consciousness; this occurs through simple metaphors and visuals so that we can have a basic appreciation for what might be occurring even though what is transpiring is quantum.

CELLULAR COMMUNICATION

From the information I had received during my channeling sessions, as well as what I had learned from various sources on how we communicate with our DNA and our cells, I decided to apply the guidance to my own situation. I reasoned that because the Innate Self is quantum, it was possible to influence my genetic code by asking my Innate Self to facilitate a correction to the instructions being provided to my cells through my quantum DNA. The Innate Self understands everything that's happening in the body and controls the messages sent to the cells. As Kryon, channeled through Lee Carroll, points out, "[w]ithout conscious direction given to your body often, your cellular structure has no boss, no instructions other than those you are born with. Now you know why we ask you to 'talk to the cells,' for the great 'listener' is the DNA!"[14]

On a daily basis, during my meditation sessions, I called on my Higher Self, Spirit, and specific spiritual entities that I am accustomed to working with to hold space for this work and to assist me with my intention. I gave permission to my Innate Self to make whatever adjustments were required to achieve my goals as a perfectly functioning biological organism. I asked my cells to release any memory they had retained, including any past or current patterns of dysfunction, misinformation, and disease. I called on my Innate Self to extract the blueprints (frequency information) for perfect stem cells (undifferentiated cells that are the templates for our genes) that were held in my quantum DNA and, in particular, those instructions that would be most beneficial for me, given my health circumstances and my conscious intention to heal. I would remind my cells that each of them contained within them this DNA blueprint for optimal and effective functioning. I encouraged my cells to release or void any previous instructions provided by my biological DNA, particularly those that were propagating an unhealthy state for me at the cellular level.

The conversations I had with my Innate Self and my cells most often included positive affirmation statements. After several sessions, my Higher Self started to step in and the most amazing statements would come up spontaneously to address my cells. Most of these were about recognizing the truth of my divinity, my cells and my body as an expression of the divine, and about my inseparable connection with the multidimensional reality that I am a part of. When we open ourselves up to the divinity within, we create limitless potential for healing and transformation to occur. I sincerely believed in this innate capacity for self-healing and regulation—I was not just trying to convince myself or my cells. I held this belief with each and every intention I established during these exercises. There was no doubt when I formulated my conscious intention for these sessions that I was going through a process of remembering this consciously and was reminding my cells of this. These cell communication sessions resembled a form of self-talk, or inner speech. I was prompting my cells and my body to recall the perfection that they once knew and could have again. In as much as we have forgotten these things when we incarnate, by design, the very process of healing and transformation is remembering this again through an elevation in consciousness and higher states of awareness of self. How could my cells not respond when they were reminded of things so fundamental to their existence and their sacredness?

Trusting in the abilities of the Innate Self as being smart and intelligent, I was confident that I did not need to be a medical expert or a scientist to know exactly what specific information would be necessary to correct some of the problems that were occurring at the cellular level. I did not need to instruct my cells directly to repair the cell structure, adjust the cell transport mechanisms, or mediate the cell signaling processes in particular ways. My intent therefore was to express my desire for change and give my cells permission to do so, but I left the specifics up to the Innate Self and quantum DNA to facilitate the response necessary. Sometimes, powerful images were revealed during these meditations, showing me the malfunctioning mechanisms of my cell receptor/effector and signaling responses, and so I would visualize a change in these to reflect proper cell functioning to support my intentions.

I talked to my cells on a daily basis for several months, continually confirming my desire to heal and transform. I expressed my gratitude for their support and for carrying me through some very difficult stretches, and I promised to, and did, do what I could to support them and care for them by looking after my body through diet, adequate rest, and what I could do at the time in the form of movement and modest exercise. I had previously learned with forays into other realms of consciousness that the more we travel a path into the unknown, the more the direction becomes known to us. I reasoned that in the same way if I reinforced my intent frequently enough, eventually the pattern of the message would surely become engrained and my cells would oblige.

In these meditative states, as always, I focused on releasing the negative energies associated with discordant thoughts and emotions and on generating a positive state in which to hold these intentions. Over time, changes to my energy field began to transpire as a result of self-work, applying the consciousness tools as well as the intuitive work and healing work I had been doing both for myself and for others. My vibration levels increased as a result. I believe the process of cellular communication began to build on itself in this way, likely via the process of entrainment, which I described earlier. When exposed to a quantum field, my cells would have theoretically entrained or adjusted themselves to the higher vibrational energies and information they contained. By virtue of our quantum nature and that of cellular communities, cells learn from each other to resonate to the new information contained in a higher energetic state. In a quantum way, if I could talk to my cells, then I could reasonably assume that they could, in turn, talk to each other and share this information. This was an exciting and very promising prospect in terms of the potential for healing.

Some of my clients ask me to write them a script or tell them what to say to their cells, and so I have provided an example in the appendix. However, it is important to remember that when the Innate Self is involved in the process of communicating with our DNA or translating the specific energies contained in the quantum DNA for utilization in our biological functioning, they are the subject matter experts. The Innate Self understands and knows what we need—no matter how specific our instructions are or exactly what we say. We don't need to worry about "getting it right," about what precisely is wrong with us at a cellular or genetic level, or how sick we are. As long as a genuine intention is held during this exercise, the Innate understands. Our quantum DNA recognizes the energy behind our thoughts and emotions that comprises our conscious intent, not the specific language of instructions that our words make. It is the body's intelligent quantum energy, provided through our conscious-ness and Innate Self, that knows what is wrong and knows how to alter cellular operations to repair, regenerate, and resume a healthier state.

MINING OR RECALIBRATING THE AKASH

As previously indicated, our Akashic Records (Akash) are stored in the crystalline structure of our quantum DNA as memory or, in other words, as a vibration, which is effectively a distribution of frequencies. In one of my meditations, when asking for clarification on the subject, a very simple metaphor was provided to explain this concept. I was shown a drawer containing huge stacks of paper, representing my soul's Akashic Records, ordered throughout time. At certain intervals there were colored tabs or markers inserted between the pages. The arrange-ment of my records looked rather like a filing system or a catalog of various energetic patterns and designs created as a result of the mental, emotional, and spiritual energy I had generated in response to my past and present life experiences. Alterations in the frequency pattern were shown as piles of paper becoming compressed or squished together; missing frequencies or gaps were shown as some of the sheets of paper being crumpled and thrown out. This is consistent with the original premise that incoherent patterns of energy are created when all frequen-cies in the spectral range are not represented or participating. Despite what I had learned about the influence of thoughts, emotions, and genetic coding at the soul level on the energetic patterns represented in our personal quantum field, this was new insight. From this, I realized that we also have the choice to change this energy at will. This means we can rewrite many of our attributes at will and by choice, erasing the negative effects of bad habits, beliefs, and past trauma, creating lasting change in both our personalities and our health. DNA, therefore, can be altered, thus affecting how we manifest health and wellness and even our character by substituting different frequencies within the Akash using conscious intent. This effectively constitutes a recalibration of the frequencies (information) held within the Akash, which increases the vibration and improves coherence and electrical flow in our fields, ultimately resulting in enhanced communication with our DNA.

This means we can rewrite many of our attributes at will and by choice, erasing the negative effects of bad habits, beliefs, and past trauma, creating lasting change in both our personalities and our health.

This was a critical turning point in my own healing when I was advised that I was to "mine my Akash." The beauty of our quantumness is that we essentially are our past, present, and our future in any given moment. Since our Akashic Records contain past energies and all of the wisdom associated with that past experience, we can access or "mine" aspects from the past, pull them forward, and replace our current energies with more desirable and beneficial ones from the past. Part of our soul's journey, as I have mentioned, is that when we enter a new incarnation, we are not a new entity, we have simply forgotten who we really are. We have acquired and learned many things over the course of the multitude of expressions we have undertaken as a soul, and we can access positive attributes of ourselves from the past if we so choose. The Akashic Records contain the attributes we need for self-mastery.[15] It contains every strength, talent, or positive attribute that we possessed at one time or another, even if we do not exhibit these in our current life. We can activate their energies and apply these to our current attributes, which in turn activates our quantum DNA to bring about healing, transformation, and the manifestation of our highest potential.

Thus, the energy from our Akash is changeable. However, because one of the fundamental laws of spirituality and humanity is free will, changing these cannot be done unless we exercise this free will as conscious choice.

> Everything you have is changeable, right down to the diseases you carry in your blood. It's only the Akash. . . . It's part of your DNA so it belongs to you . . . if the storehouse of who you used to be, which is contained in your own DNA, included a beautiful, young, healthy Human being, it is therefore, still there![16]

Kryon says that much of the DNA (and therefore our Akash) is just data ready to be changed if we so choose and that what we were born with doesn't matter. The DNA energetic patterns that are part of past-life templates can be rewritten by mining our Akash.[17] We can shift our biology and our genetic coding in this way when we change or alter our quantum DNA frequencies.

> **The DNA energetic patterns that are part of past-life templates can be rewritten by mining our Akash. We can shift our biology and our genetic coding in this way when we change or alter our quantum DNA frequencies.**

As a practitioner, I have performed a Shamanic technique known as "soul contracts" on some of my clients, which I believe is analogous to mining our Akash. Similar to soul programs, a contract can lock us into very deep-seated beliefs that can place a filter on perceptions of our reality and create many problems for us, including making us ill. It is a method of soul healing in which the energy of a story from the past, believed to be contributing to or causing a particular disease or challenge in a person's life, is brought forward. Essentially, the script to the story is then rewritten, and the energy is changed when the person agrees to a different ending, usually one that is offered by Spirit and then accepted by the person. In my case, during a session with my own practitioner employing this same method, I was shown an image of myself sitting at a desk looking over a complete record I had kept of what every single person in my life thought of me. In reality, as I have mentioned, I experienced difficulty in the past making decisions, taking responsibility for things, and making changes in my life. This was due to the irrational fear that had consumed me because I was so worried about how everyone was judging and perceiving me. In many ways, this fear had become paralyzing and very self-limiting. The new scenario was presented to me in which I was provided with a completely blank set of pages, and I was free to choose what I felt about my own self, uninfluenced by others. I later went on to use this technique in my own practice, with many beautiful soul contract endings rewritten for my clients, with very positive results in their energy fields and their lives.

Substitution of energies in our Akash means that we maintain the overall balance of energies through an exchange process. We void the energies that do not serve us in this life or that we do not wish to have by substituting them for those from the past that do. Through our Higher Self and Innate Self, we give permission to activate those energies in our quantum DNA that will help us heal and accomplish our life's purpose.

It's not that you're going into the DNA and getting something different to paste upon you. Actually, it's an exchange, one for another. . . . For the DNA claims everything that you are. What you are doing is exchanging attributes . . . putting into the record what doesn't suit your energy and claiming the things that do. You own them all.[18]

The past cannot be erased during this substitution and remains there with all of its memories. However, there is an opportunity for us to change how we might remember or respond to the past. If, for example, we are influenced in a negative way from a past life in which there was trauma or a horrific event, we can mine the Akash, pulling forward the energy of peace or resilience from a past life in which there was no trauma or suffering.

In addition, Kryon also says in the new energy (since the year 2013) many will start to use these quantum Akashic tools. In addition to this method of mining the Akash, there is also the concept of quantum Akashic Inheritance. He says that this date marks the beginning of humanity's ability to remember "original galactic ancestor knowledge and is open to the oldest souls, only after full realization of the God inside."[19]

You can well imagine the possibilities and implications of this astounding piece of information. The self-healing capability we possess seemed very apparent with the realization that I could at will change the data within my own quantum DNA, through my Akashic Records, to manifest results on all levels of my being. I was no longer fearful of what I might find out about myself or afraid of change if it meant potential changes of this magnitude.

I began in earnest, through regular meditation sessions and establishing specific conscious intentions, to work with substituting frequencies in my Akash to create a completely healthy, vital, and disease-free state. On a daily basis, I called upon my Higher Self, Spirit, the spiritual entities I work with, as well as my Innate Self, to assist me by pulling forward energies from the past and applying them to my quantum DNA. The old energies responsible for my disease were replaced with these new ones, originating from times when I was perfectly healthy and every single cell in my body was functioning optimally and without error. When we establish a pure intention to mine the Akash, it will trigger the Innate Self to go and acquire the appropriate frequencies that are needed.[20] I asked for energies to be pulled forward from past circumstances in which there was no disease or medical condition of any sort, when I was completely absent of any pain. I requested energies from when there was absolutely no physical impairment, no physiological or biological dysfunction. I was also interested in manifesting many other attributes consistent with my goals as a practitioner, a writer, and a teacher. Over the course of many months, I called forward energies relating to skills as a healer, a warrior, and an orator. I focused on manifesting attributes of strength, tenacity, and confidence.

During these meditations, I was never cognizant of the particular frequencies that were being substituted. I was not made aware of specific past-life experiences from which the energies were being drawn. I did not have to put my life or my health under a microscope to list all of the attributes that weren't working for me and for which I required substitutions. I had been through a lot of those exercises already, through previous energy and soul work as well as my own Akashic Record activities, so with exception of a few particular cases where I felt it appropriate to specify, I left this up to my Innate Self to decide on my behalf.

I simply stated my conscious intention and asked my Innate Self, Higher Self, and Spirit to carry out the work, acknowledging my Innate Self's ability to know what frequencies would be appropriate and helpful for me based on that intention. I gave permission and empowered my Innate Self to integrate those energies into my being in a way that was appropriate and right for me. Using conscious intention in this way, our quantum DNA recognizes these conscious thoughts and can actually provide new information to the instruction sets of our biological DNA. I did not ask "God" to do this for me; I entrusted myself and all aspects of me including my Higher Self and Innate Self with the power to perform the task. There was no healer or practitioner required, nor someone who could perform miracles. I was doing this alone, working with multidimensional energies via my consciousness in my own personal quantum field.

A sample script used for mining the Akash is provided for those who wish to embark on this exercise alone. The script is intended as an example only—much like the cellular communication exercise, the actual specifics of the message itself and how it is communicated are less important than an intention that is genuinely expressed. Innate understands the intent, what is being asked, and what is needed. More recently, Spirit has begun to implement some of these substitutions and modifications in Akashic frequencies through me for clients during our treatment sessions, depending on their own level of conscious awareness and readiness in undertaking these exercises themselves.

10

Altering DNA and Its Effects

Re-encoding Genes for New Form and Function

The universe is a memory-filled world of constant and enduring interconnection, a world where everything informs—acts on and interacts with—everything else. We should apprehend this remarkable world with our heart as well as with our intellect . . . a vision that is imaginative but not imaginary: a poetic vision of a cosmos where nothing disappears without a trace, where all things that exist are, and remain, intrinsically and intimately interconnected.

ERVIN LASZLO[1]

RE-ENCODING GENES

Throughout the book, I have repeatedly stated that by employing the consciousness tools, it was possible to re-encode my genes. The word *encode* describes a process by which information is converted into a format that can be stored in some way, and then read and translated in order to generate a response. In the context of conventional genetics, the term implies genetic information that is encoded on our biological DNA, based on the specific nucleotide base pair sequences, that specifies instructions for the synthesis of various protein molecules. However, given what has been outlined in previous chapters, the type of information encoded on our DNA contains not only the sequencing information present on the biological, but also quantum information or light codes present as an array of frequencies imprinted on the quantum DNA as well. This creates the DNA blueprint based on this quantum holographic light information, which is then communicated to the instruction sets that comprise our biological DNA. The communication of this information by the quantum DNA and its interpretation by the biological portion results in the re-encoding or the alteration of the gene coding sequences. As mentioned, the frequencies or energy associated with our entire life's event history is recorded as memory in our Akashic Records (Akash) and makes up a portion of our quantum DNA. Not all of these frequencies or energies are appropriate and optimal for various reasons, as we have learned, and may in fact be contributing to disease, along with other undesirable consequences.

Since frequencies are essentially energetic information, through our own consciousness we can change the frequencies and therefore alter the quantum DNA information provided to our biological DNA to execute the various instructions necessary to elicit a biological response. More quantum DNA becomes activated as we make higher frequency substitutions or augmentations that are represented by the DNA blueprint. Higher frequencies mean that there is a higher vibrational energy and thus coherence present, allowing for more efficient communication of the information between the quantum and biological portions of the DNA. Re-encoding the gene means that the DNA blueprint containing all of the information for development and functioning of the body is effectively altered; it now contains this new or enhanced information, and the information that may predispose us to disease has been removed. Through this process, we have accessed and activated quantum memory information that reminds our body and our cells how they really work to combat and prevent disease and maintain health. This is nothing short of remarkable and represents an immense opportunity for those battling with disease to support their own healing, as I had done.

My channels indicate that during the process of re-encoding our genes and in the presence of these higher frequency quantum energies, there is a complicated process in which the magnetic characteristics of the DNA actually shift. Magnetic field mechanisms are the means by which quantum information is attracted and imprinted on our DNA. There are also specific "transition frequencies" that change and result in small shifts in the energy levels of the DNA molecule. The frequency arrays become more ordered (coherent), which essentially provides more stable and enduring gene encoding arrangements. Ultimately, these prescribe better instructions and prioritization of tasks in the body, such as optimal cellular functioning, repair, and regeneration via the biological instruction sets than what might have been previously present during disease states.

It was also indicated to me that during the re-encoding process, there is a movement toward what was described as *desiccation,* a term that means the removal of water by chemical or physical means. DNA assumes different conformational structures and geometry depending on water activity. Scientific evidence suggests that "the precise DNA structure depends on specific amounts of water surrounding the molecule."[2] The restructuring of water alters energetic patterns that are held in the water and plays a role in the transmission and storage of genetic information. Presumably, when the water content is lessened and it becomes restructured through desiccation, the structural orientation of the DNA changes and possibly unfurls for re-encoding purposes. This may in part be due to the altered strengths of the bonds between the helix structure and its base pairs. In addition, for the gene to be re-encoded, the protective water sheath surrounding the DNA structure has to be removed to expose the surface of the DNA so that it can access this new information. This could be to facilitate the exposure of the ten invisible strands of multidimensional DNA that exist in addition to the two visible physical strands, and that become activated through the receipt of this new quantum information. As a result, the DNA blueprint changes. In order for the new instructions encoded in the DNA to manifest in the body, they would then go through the normal DNA replication process. This involves the messenger RNA copying the instructions from the cleaved DNA strand and then transcribing it into amino acids, which are the building blocks that create form and function in the body.

EVIDENCE OF CHANGE

The consciousness tools I have described are really quantum transactions dealing with energy and consciousness that occur in a nonlinear, multidimensional kind of way. Most of the changes occurred at the energetic, quantum DNA level and cellular level. Because science currently has no way of measuring these nonphysical aspects of our quantum DNA and our consciousness, we have little proof of their existence, as is the case with all other quantum attributes studied by science. Until this changes, we can only observe the transformation they instill in us at all levels—emotionally, mentally, spiritually, and physically. Over the course of the year that I worked extensively with the consciousness tools, I noticed a dramatic shift in my healing progression as well as tangible changes that I attributed to these activities including the following:

- Improvement in or elimination of physical health conditions— eradication of tumors and cancer cells, enhanced healing of damaged tissue and injuries, improved metabolic function (digestion, cellular absorption), stimulation of detoxification process
- Improvement in or elimination of physical symptoms—less pain and discomfort, less inflammation and nerve response (requiring

less medication to abate symptoms), less stiffness in spine and more mobility, disappearance of feeling of overall malaise

- Improvement in energy levels, less fatigue, improved strength and stamina, change in activity levels and exercise
- Increasing speed of recovery after physical interventions, periodic inflammatory, or neuropathic episodes
- Improvement in quality of life and focus, level of engagement, activities, and relationships
- Change in thoughts and emotions—more positive outlook, more positive emotions including acceptance, contentment, patience, compassion, and love; fewer negative emotions such as fear, anger, and judgment; increased mental clarity
- Change in perception of self-limitations, more optimism about future possibilities and manifesting changes at all levels
- Ability to surrender and let go
- Deepening sense of spiritual connectedness and sense of self, expanded consciousness

Toward the beginning of my work with my first natural healing arts practitioner, she conducted what is referred to as an "internal viewing" assessment. As an exceptionally capable healer and intuitive, using her inner sight, she views the physical body as though with x-ray vision, just as my subsequent practitioner could. She traveled through my body like a tiny submarine with a camera attached, reporting her observations and any apparent abnormalities. She noted the iliopsoas muscle group that attaches to the spine at the T12 vertebra and areas on the lumbar spine did not look healthy. The muscle fibers appeared to be loose and partially detached in this area, with some abnormality seen in the fibers themselves. The psoas major and minor muscles travel from the front of the lumbar spinal vertebrae, diagonally down through the abdomen, beneath the intestines to attach on the front of the femur (thighbone) just to the inside of the hip joint. The iliacus muscle lines the inside of the ilium, or pelvic bone, then feeds into the common tendon with the major and minor psoas. The tendon that joins them was completely in the wrong position. My practitioner commented on the poor quality of the psoas muscle tissue in this area, likely indicative of necrosis, or oxidative or vascular compromise, similar to the T12 insertion area, which also exhibited abnormal honeycomb-like structures in some areas. She observed herniated discs in the cervical, thoracic, and lumbar spine as well as what she thought was incorrect positioning and functioning of many nerves along the thoracic and lumbar spine. The nerves emanating from thoracic vertebra T8, where I had received radiation for the spinal tumor, also appeared abnormal, and she sensed that they were unable to conduct nerve signals adequately. Finally, there was an osteophyte (bone chip) on the top of my left femoral head and a synovial lesion, which she described as a 2-inch-long, one-third of an inch thick, spongy, gel-like mass inside my left hip cavity itself. Fortunately, I have improved function in most of these areas, and in the hip, pelvic, and sacroiliac regions in particular, where my recovery is very apparent. I no longer experience any uncomfortable sensations or pain around the thoracic vertebra T8 nor with my psoas muscle.

Once my work with consciousness tools began in earnest, regular visits to my practitioner revealed some interesting changes at an energetic level. After the removal of my DNA markers and associated soul patterns, during an appointment for Chinese Five Element energy work and meridian balancing, my practitioner (who was not involved in the DNA marker and pattern work and therefore had no preconceived bias) noted with surprise that my energetic signature had completely changed. She had worked with me on a weekly basis for over three years by that time and was very familiar with the character of my meridian pulses as well as the look and feel of my subtle energy body. For her to say that I now felt like a completely different person on an energetic level was definitely significant. When I first began to see her, she described my pulses as being indicative of an almost frenetic or chaotic chi (life force), whereas now she described them as being much more orderly and calm. This undoubtedly was a sign of increasing energetic coherence within my personal quantum field and was extremely encouraging. On several occasions, she was able to detect a perceptible increase in my overall vibration, which she described as an upward shift in my harmonics. I believe that my sound and breath work had a significant impact in this regard. I was very pleased.

Other notable changes included a complete shift in the electrical flow through my body. When I first began work with my second practitioner, my physical body was in such a depleted state that I was unable to hold any appreciable charge. Initially, and though I had experienced some improvements through an increase in vibration, she said I was still "pocketing these transcendent, high vibration states." I could not hold this state consistently all of the time. Over the course of several months—aided by clearing, adjustments to my field energy, and supplements—this changed dramatically and my electromagnetic field strengthened immeasurably. With the activation of remaining points on my subtle energetic bodies, I began to open up to full-streaming consciousness and a much more efficient and faster exchange of information between my physical body and my light body.

After about six months, I was informed that my cellular response was improving. Less than a year later, I was told through a channel that I had experienced a significant shift in my DNA and cellular matrices. When I heard this, at first it was hard to believe that I had actually been able to influence healing in my body in this way and that I was out of immediate danger. The downward spiral of physiological dysfunction and disease had been impeded; my health was taking a turn for the better. I (through Spirit, my Innate, and Higher Self) had promoted healing through the soul work and the consciousness tools I had employed. Through my own efforts, by activating and re-encoding my DNA, the fact that I had invoked a more appropriate cellular response to facilitate proper repair and regeneration mechanisms in the tissue, blood, and bone to help restore normal function to my body seemed nothing short of miraculous. I had actually achieved results beyond what even I thought was truly possible. Although the journey had been long and oftentimes fraught with terrible symptoms and compromise, I felt exonerated and was anxious to help others heal in the same way.

DNA EFFICIENCY AND ACTIVATION

DNA efficiency is a measure of the degree to which our spiritual and biological DNA communicate with each other. As we activate more DNA, a higher state of consciousness results. This increases our vibration level (coherence) and, thus, the DNA efficiency or the extent to which these two parts of our DNA communicate effectively. When DNA starts to work at higher efficiency, the Higher Self, Innate Self, and consciousness begin to work as a team, providing better instructions to our bodies to create a more aware and healthy state. As we have learned, consciousness is the big driver in influencing what we manifest, and if we reflect on where we are as a human species—the ongoing wars and unrest, socioeconomic problems, and the prevalence of disease and illness in all cultures, it might be fair to conclude that we have not exactly lived up to our fullest potential. It appears as though we have actually devolved as a species, away from the potential that has been instilled in us. Over time, generation after generation, we have become separate from the quantum aspects of our DNA, of ourselves, and our own divinity—losing our intuition and ability to know how to work with and heal our bodies, among other things. Part of this is intentional and by design, representing the soul's "Earth journey" and our goal to evolve as a species by expanding our consciousness so as to remember these important aspects of who we are. It has been said that presently most people, with the exception of those that are more consciously aware or spiritually awakened, have DNA efficiencies of 30 percent. This means that a large portion of our DNA is not functioning as it was designed to do. When DNA is working at 100 percent, we "have the empowerment of the creator fully manifested within the Human Being. The efficiency factor is not chemical, but informational."[3]

Therefore, poor communication between our quantum DNA, the

memory held within the crystalline structure of our DNA, and the instructions that reside within our biological DNA is the only thing that stands between us and perfect health.[4] Our magnetic environment (overlapping magnetic fields) and the mechanism of information transfer via electrical impulse previously described is what enables the communication between the two parts of our DNA to take place. Our bodies and our cells have forgotten how to repair and regenerate themselves. We are vulnerable to disease because, at a very deep level, we have forgotten how this works. At lower levels of DNA efficiency, much of the encoding in our genes is not working, since it has no information from the crystalline structure and the memory that is held there to help the DNA chemistry remember how it operates. As the memory transmission is increased to the instruction sets through our consciousness, more DNA is activated and the body responds.[5] It is the Innate Self in conjunction with the DNA that decides what portion of the DNA is activated, not the healer or the individual. Once triggered with the expression of intent as described, the gene formats and configures itself in ways it knows are needed.[6] The quantum DNA recognizes the intent or conscious thought and gives instructions to the biological portion of the DNA to change or adjust.

Once triggered with the expression of intent as described, the gene formats and configures itself in ways it knows are needed. The quantum DNA recognizes the intent or conscious thought and gives instructions to the biological portion of the DNA to change or adjust.

Every cell of the human body is designed for self-diagnostics and to know whether it is correct or out of balance with the whole; but when our DNA efficiency is low, much of this information is hidden from it. When more quantum information can be transmitted to our cells in an efficient manner, the cells become fully intelligent.[7] They are able to recognize when they are out of balance and what cells are not functioning properly. The cells exercise their own self-management strategy to maintain balance by eliminating the unhealthy cells through normal mechanisms such as apoptosis; they regenerate only healthy ones. It is clear that given this capability, if our DNA efficiency is high, many diseases including more serious ones like cancer, simply would not exist. As our DNA efficiency increases, we are activating a greater portion of our quantum DNA, thereby raising our consciousness. We begin to awaken to the truth of who we are and our innate capacity to heal. Thus, most gifted healers, meditators, and spiritually awakened individuals would theoretically exhibit higher DNA efficiency.

> **It is clear that given this capability, if our DNA efficiency is high, many diseases including more serious ones like cancer, simply would not exist.**

As we have seen, the body is designed to heal, but it does this by responding to quantum energies that are communicated via our consciousness. Healing is not controlled by chemistry; it is controlled by quantum information, but we have to purposefully communicate this new information to it, through our intent. In this way, we are expanding our own consciousness. It is said that this can actually "alter the magnetic portions of the cellular frame, creating a kind of healing that is not understood . . . and is not chemical."[8] This aspect of our DNA needs to be addressed daily, until the misinformation is no longer propagated.

The process of re-encoding genes does not reverse itself, and so once our DNA is activated, it stays that way. Having now achieved higher DNA efficiency levels, I have been able to release any fear about the return of any cancer or the possibility that new tumors or other issues may surface for any reason known to me at this time. Even if they did, I feel confident that they could also be influenced for a better outcome by the means I have described.

I began to ask about my DNA efficiency in order to gauge my progress on a regular basis as I conducted these consciousness exercises. I would determine the level I received during my channels, using a pendulum and a number chart. Pendulums are a type of divination tool, and when used under these circumstances, are a means of determining our ideomotor (subconscious reflexive) response or answer to specific questions that are posed. I believe this is actually our Innate Self working through the pendulum to provide a response, in the same way that muscle testing provides feedback from our Innate Self. The first time I measured it, my efficiency was on the low side. Over the course of about six months or more, this increased to a significantly higher level, relatively speaking. I surmised that the increase I eventually achieved was attributed to a shift in my DNA, through the various means that follow:

- Consistently embodying the intention to heal in my practices and daily life
- Embracing a desire to be present in and inhabit my physical body, despite the physical symptoms
- Harmonizing my personal quantum field and clearing discordant energies driven by programs of the soul and subconscious mind
- Increasing my vibration through sound and breath, meditation, conscious awareness, and physical body support

- Communicating with my cells and DNA
- Mining my Akash, substituting frequencies, and bringing forward past energies associated with a healthy state and more desirable attributes

REGENERATION AND REPAIR

When it is possible to begin to heal as I had by completely altering my cellular matrices and DNA, initially the *how* seemed far less important to me. I was so overjoyed with the improvement in my condition and a dissipation in my terrible symptoms, living more freely and with less compromise and infirmity after so many years, that it did not seem to matter as much. If my healing had been called a miracle instead of quantum, most would simply accept the mystery of the event and be happy with the results.

However, in order to provide an explanation to others so they could understand, as well as to encourage them to follow a similar approach to healing, through my own intuitive abilities and the process of inquiry, I was provided with an explanation of much of what had occurred. When I inquired through my channels about what was happening as result of these exercises, they indicated a modulation in frequencies was underway and a process of harmonization in my field was occurring, so that the DNA could be altered and new DNA activated. They described how through the various intentions I had established, certain light frequencies had been accessed from a complete library or catalog of frequencies available to me from multidimensional origins. These frequencies were adjusting and augmenting existing light patterns that make up the DNA blueprint. This newly altered DNA information was being energetically communicated, received, and interpreted by my cells via the instruction sets on my biological DNA by the mechanisms described previously. As a result of this DNA activation, the genes were being re-encoded to produce a more favorable and healthy response in the body.

About six months after I began working with the consciousness tools, I understood that there were still some energetic anomalies that remained in my field and that these required some adjustments, so I continued on with the exercises. At that time, through my channels, I was informed that the process of information transference via inductance (overlapping of quantum fields of information) was underway, and that the physical DNA was beginning to unfurl in preparation to receive this new information. The quantum light information was essentially being implemented upon the DNA structure. In response to this, the "perturbations," as they referred to them, meaning the process by which genetic mutations are created and propagated from cell to cell during the cell division and replication process, began to slow down, eventually stopping altogether not long afterward. Now that the frequencies of the DNA markers had been adjusted and higher and more positive frequencies were being drawn in from my Akash and substituted for old ones, consistency and coherence was beginning to develop in my field and in the quantum holographic light patterns being communicated. I was absolutely amazed and quite humbled to learn of the positive impact my consciousness work was having at a cellular and genetic level—without any other form of physical intervention or assistance. It was then that I began to reflect more seriously on the enormity of this outcome and its implications for healing and potentially the eradication of chronic and incurable disease by these means for others.

A shift in my DNA was definitely occurring, and I was reminded of the need to continue focusing on devising purposeful intentions to bring about the necessary changes in my DNA and at the cellular level. I was advised that "masterful intention makes and organizes matter" and that this masterful intention was "imbued with light," constituting the frequencies needed for the cellular and DNA transformation to occur. Truly, conscious intent can manifest changes, even in the physical realm. When I asked what I could do to support what was happening, I was told I needed to "hold the charge" and "hold the pieces together in the pattern." I mentioned earlier that it is important to ensure our electromagnetic field is strong so that our cells' electrical properties are conducive to the transmission of quantum genetic information (holographic light patterns) that is imprinted on our DNA. Thus, I continued to focus on the aspects of my daily practice centered on raising and maintaining my physical and field vibration at a high level. These included the sound and breath work, meditation, focusing on positive thoughts and emotions, as well as adhering to a clean and healthy diet. Limiting the intake of prescription medications, which also lower vibrational energy, as well as harmonizing those that I still required to alleviate extreme symptoms from time to time within my field, was also necessary. This is akin to what is commonly referred to as "holding the light" by promoting good energetic balance (pattern consistency) and flow, as well as maintaining a state of harmony at a high level of vibration.

I was curious about how my genes were being altered as a result of the change in frequencies from the consciousness tools I was working with. The response I received was that "changes were being excised in order of importance" and included alterations to attributes and expression previously being solely dictated by the instructions from my biological DNA. My DNA and Innate Self were undoubtedly governing the healing process by prioritizing and implementing changes that were appropriate for me. My channels indicated there were changes in what they called "signaling patterns" and a "reassembly of quanta." Recall from the mechanisms described earlier, genetic information is conveyed from multidimensional origins via electrical impulses containing quantum particles, transported through quantum fields by harmonic oscillations. I assumed from this that some of the genetic coding information was being altered as well as the means by which the information was transmitted or enhanced in some way. Cellular and DNA changes followed suit.

I continued to ask for status updates in my channeling sessions, and after several months, I was informed that normal energetic forces were present, cellular functioning was returning to normal, and my toxic load had decreased. Improvements in the energetic state and electrical flow within my personal quantum field were beginning to create effects at the cellular level via the information provided in the revised DNA blueprint. The electrical potential of the cell membranes was transitioning to a more electropositive state, "settling the contractions" (cell structure collapse). As the cell membranes began to regain structure and maintain capacitance, membrane permeability improved, enabling better transport of nutrients across the membrane as well as cell signaling. Improved intracellular communication followed as normal mechanisms of repair, regeneration, and function were instituted with the energetic improvements. Still, I was advised that the frequencies were not yet stable, and I was told that my cell shape, in other words, the conformational shapes in the cytoskeletal structure or cell matrix, still required adjustment for optimum functioning in order to hold the light. I was informed that the cellular matrices needed to expand further from their collapsed state, to allow for enhanced electrical flow and further change. And so, I continued with my daily practice of working with the consciousness tools.

My vibration increased steadily over the following weeks as a result of my daily consciousness work. As previously indicated, there is a threshold capacitance necessary for optimal electrical conductivity, and thus normal biological functioning. Accordingly, the vibration has to be sufficient for the gaps in transmission to be closed so that a closed electrical circuit can be maintained. By mining my Akash, and the sound and breath sessions in particular, higher and more appropriate frequencies were being applied to my DNA and cells and also retained through my ever strengthening electromagnetic field.

In less than six months, my channels began to indicate that the energetic distortions in my personal quantum field were declining and more harmony was beginning to develop. This state of harmony was described as a "closed cadence" condition, which by definition is the strongest type of harmony that exists and is a harmonic configuration that creates resolution or completion in a "structurally defining moment."[9] Various cellular functioning tasks require not only a certain level of vibrational energy to achieve optimal capacitance, but also a specific range of frequencies in the spectrum of light to do the job. Similar or different frequencies (colors) combine to make harmonic frequencies that make up light patterns. At any frequency other than a harmonic frequency, the resulting disturbance creates irregular and nonrepeating patterns. The state of energetic discord that was present initially at the cellular and genetic level was influenced by this newer state of harmonic accord, bringing existing frequencies into attunement or, in other words, into a more harmonious and responsive state. Fewer frequency anomalies were said to be present, and the light patterns were being updated as well as becoming more organized and coherent. Attunement can only occur with a specific combination of both low and high frequencies. A spectrum of harmonic frequencies contains sounds of varying speed. Varying speeds of sound in turn result in friction due to opposing forces, which creates entropy. *Entropy* is defined as "the average amount of information contained in each message." This implies that the harmony was enhancing the amount of quantum information available to activate the DNA and revise the DNA blueprint information so that it could be communicated to induce an appropriate cellular and genetic response.

During disease processes, physical changes to DNA occur in two ways, either by mutation or damage. Free nucleotides or bases—guanine (G), adenine (A), thymine (T), or cytosine (C)—are available to bond with the nucleotides that exist along the exposed backbone of the DNA strand during the replication process. According to proper base pairing rules, A bonds with T (or T with A), and C bonds with G (or G with C). Under suboptimal conditions and in the presence of triggers for disease, mutations occur when the rules are not followed and incorrect base pairing occurs (such as A with C or G). These gene sequencing abnormalities are then copied when a cell divides and replicates. Once they occur, mutations cannot be repaired because enzymes that activate protein function and regulation repair mechanisms do not recognize altered base sequences. Physical abnormalities may occur in DNA in the form of broken or damaged chromosomes. Normally, damage due to environmental factors and normal metabolic processes occurs on a continuous basis. However, repair mechanisms are sometimes impaired, particularly when cells have accumulated a large amount of DNA damage. Unregulated cell division and resulting tumor formation, cell death (*apoptosis*), or cell dormancy (*senescence*) are all indications that DNA is unable to perform effective repair processes, as was seen in my case. Changes in chemistry involving alteration to the bases through chemical processes such as oxidation, alkylation, or hydrolysis or the bonding of foreign chemicals (called *adducts*) to the DNA, disrupt and damage its helical structure. This can create single or double breaks in the DNA strands, crosslinking between incorrect bases, or mismatching of bases in which the wrong base is stitched into place in a newly formed DNA strand or a base is skipped in the matching of the base ends to each other.[10]

In addition to the cessation of the deleterious mutation process that had occurred some months ago, my channels indicated that as a result of the improvements in the cell structure and function, as well as the DNA activation, a number of DNA repair mechanisms were now taking place. A change in the quantum information and re-encoding of the genes had initiated a chemical response in the body to prompt DNA repair. Mismatched base repairs were described as being operational and likely included a number of possible mechanisms. My channels indicated that "correct end matching" was occurring as well as the "binding of proteins." Changes in cellular signaling can activate a repair response in which specific proteins bind to the DNA. This induces the transcription of repair genes "allowing for further signal induction, inhibition of cell division, and an increase in the levels of proteins responsible for damage processing."[11] In all likelihood, proteins were being generated that were able to detect the mismatch and recruit enzymes, which in turn cleaved damaged areas of the strands. Broken nucleobases are joined together by enzymes that catalyze the formation of a special bond between the DNA backbone and the nucleotide. Damaged bases may also be removed and replaced with a base found on the other undamaged complementary DNA strand as part of the repair process. The integrity and accessibility of the information contained in the biological instructions sets, initially corrupted through DNA damage, was thereby improved, ultimately resulting in a return to a state of health.

After many long years of feeling poorly, of pain and discomfort and repeated attempts to stave off my inevitable demise, my healing journey was in full swing and my struggle was finally over. In retrospect, committing about thirty to forty-five minutes per day for a period of less than twelve months (and only six of those intensely) to perform the consciousness exercises needed to achieve this level of influence on my body seems infinitesimally small in comparison to the length of time that I was actually really ill and feeling compromised. We live in a world of immediacy and are often looking for instant fixes for lifelong problems, or for someone to fix them for us, but all in all, the time it took for me to initiate healing was incredibly fast when I consider how severely ill I was. Spirit told me afterward that given the nature of the cellular disorder and severity of my condition, had I chosen to receive radiation or chemotherapy or had I pushed for shoulder surgery earlier, the outcome would definitely not have been in my favor, without the contribution of my own efforts to the healing process. I was applauded for my level of focus and dedication to the task of healing. I thought to myself in response, how could I not if I wanted some semblance of quality in my life and wanted to stay alive? Those who are less inclined to help themselves, give themselves permission to heal, or who succumb to the fear about disease and its consequences (which is not real), may very likely miss the powerful opportunity that an approach such as mine clearly represents.

11

Quantum Information as Our Greatest Resource

In essence, DNA electrodynamics determines everything living! And those who control it are, likewise, divinely empowered.

LEONARD HOROWITZ[1]

What has been presented here has demonstrated the profound connection and interaction we have with quantum fields of information and the potential this holds in healing even the most serious diseases, through our consciousness and our DNA. As we have seen, the universal Akashic Field provides an infinite source of sound and light information that shapes all of life and can be utilized to effect remarkable changes in our bodies at the cellular and genetic level. It is truly our greatest resource and holds incredible promise in this regard. The fact that nonlocal quantum holographic patterns of light holding this information are projected and imprinted on physical DNA and are what gives rise to our physical form and function is truly remarkable. As Leonard Horowitz points out, "sound and electrical frequency patterns interacting with DNA encode structure, including biofields . . . or morphogenetic fields" by acting as "field guides to flowing matter and energy."[2] DNA is able to process this information by receiving and transducing these signals in a way that defines our cellular structure, function, and genetic response. "This process of reading and writing the very matter of our being manifests from the genome's associative holographic memory in conjunction with its quantum nonlocality. Rapid transmission of genetic information and gene expression unite the organism as a holistic entity embedded in the larger [environmental/universal] Whole."[3]

Therefore, we are co-creators of our own form and function and what we manifest in our physical bodies through our DNA's translation of the quantum holographic information contained within our personal quantum field, the Merkaba. Here "resides the fundamental basis of your structure and your sense of self and external environment, including your health and disease in both your physiological and psychological being. Your disease structures are incorporated within it. It is here, at this level of your being where fundamental healing and physical-psychic restructuring occur."[4] Ultimately, it is the information contained in our DNA blueprint, influenced primarily by quantum information, that is the progenitor of all life—our biological genes—and is the ultimate controller of gene function, for both coding and expression purposes.

> **Ultimately, it is the information contained in our DNA blueprint, influenced primarily by quantum information, that is the progenitor of all life—our biological genes—and is the ultimate controller of gene function, for both coding and expression purposes.**

Clearly, we are much more than what science can currently measure. When we consider that our quantum DNA has the ability to inform as well as reinform the instruction sets contained in our biological DNA and re-encode the gene, we can see that our bodies are capable of healing beyond what anyone thought possible, without physical intervention. It's the 95 percent of each one of us that cannot be seen that has a more powerful influence over our physical bodies and our health than perhaps any current form of medicine or healing. Understanding the dynamics of the soul and our quantum, spiritual inheritance and how this essential and causal part of us is represented in this invisible portion of our DNA, as well as its impact on our health cannot be dismissed when we see its profound effects. By design, we are sophisticated biological organisms, capable of communicating with greater fields of intelligence that are available to us for self-regulation and healing, in a beautifully simple way. Through our consciousness, we are actually in control of what we allow into our own personal quantum field of information. When we know how to access this information and work with it, we manifest dramatic and seemingly impossible changes in ourselves and our health, as I have personally demonstrated. The bridge our consciousness creates between us and these universal quantum holographic fields of information connects us to our own ability to restore the whole when its components have become broken or dysfunctional to the point of disease. Through our own consciousness, we can revise the information in our own fields that is required for the repair, reassembly, and regeneration of our physical form and function. Our DNA, therefore, should not be viewed as a limitation but an asset we can use to achieve these results. It is possibly the greatest gift to humanity yet—it provides each of us with an opportunity, through our conscious intention, to create health and wellness within by activating the positive potentials held within our DNA.

Illness is the beacon that points us in the direction of harmony with the forces of the universe within us and around us. It is purposeful and contains potential meaning to those willing to tune in to its messages. The direction toward cure is the same as the path toward greater awareness, higher consciousness, and personal fulfillment. . . . Our illness is our model for healing. . . . Disease contains within it the potentiality of cure.[5]

Given what is currently understood about genetics, the emphasis to date has been on influencing our genetic expression by mediating the effects of our environment. Recently, genetic testing has been made accessible to the greater public. While genome characterization may be helpful in confirming disease diagnoses, identifying the propensity for potential disease, or for developing proper preventive or management strategies for disease, it can also be detrimental to our progress. It can encourage the belief that many diseases are incurable and that there are no real solutions to this predicament. There is enormous pressure placed on practitioners and health care systems by those who develop expectations for quick fix solutions, cures, and answers that are focused on addressing the fallout from the apparent fate that their genes have delivered them. However, the effect that good lifestyle choices such as diet, exercise, and mind-body therapies can have on enhancing health given our genetic history and tendencies, as a preventive measure and influencing our genetic expression, certainly cannot be discredited. By limiting exposure to environmental triggers such as toxins, heavy metals, or radiation, the risk of contracting many diseases can be minimized.

Pharmaceuticals and other medical treatments, including prospective gene therapies and genetic re-engineering approaches, are similarly focused on physical means of influencing our genetic expression. There are, of course, risks and side effects associated with many of these invasive procedures and treatment options, not to mention costs. While these may have some effect, in all cases they are targeting our genes as though they were no more than simply biological instruction sets that can be influenced physically. They do not deal with the root of the problem. Instead, these approaches involve the manipulation of our bodies and biology through chemical or mechanical means, rather than working with the energetic information that truly defines our form and function in the first place. They ignore the part of our DNA that has the most powerful influence and focus solely on the physical portion that threatens to keep us as biological organisms separate from the multidimensional sources of information that are so vital to our health and the potential elimination of disease.

We have seen that true genetic coding is the result of the combination of both quantum and biological influences. We cannot distance ourselves from the intricate relationship we share with our multidimensional, quantum fields of information and the answers they provide for healing through our consciousness and DNA. Thus, the solution clearly lies in a nonphysical, nonlinear quantum approach that addresses our states of quantum energy impoverishment and imbalance. The future goes beyond simply an ability to influence our genetic expression and the many approaches offered by science to this end, toward one in which others will be able to successfully re-encode our genes entirely. Based on the guidance I have received and my own personal experience in conjunction with the scientific and spiritual evidence that exists today, this will most likely be achieved by methodologies that involve consciousness, devices and instrumentation that use quantum energy technology, as well as targeted frequencies that are capable of altering the quantum information provided to the biological gene's instruction sets.

The importance of the mind-body-spirit connection is becoming more universally accepted and is being integrated into conventional and alternative medicine disease diagnosis and treatment regimens more than ever before. Holistic vibrational energy medicine therapies designed to remove blocks and impediments to energy flow and facilitate coherence and harmony in our personal energy fields have provided the foundation for the next evolutionary step in healing, which involves working with energy in more complicated ways. My channels and personal work in this regard have demonstrated that it is possible to access and relay multidimensional frequencies that can then be applied to our personal quantum fields and our DNA to heal and to address, as well as potentially eradicate, serious disease and ultimately re-encode our genes. Missing frequencies or frequencies that are appropriate in completing the energetic pattern information required for optimal health and biological functioning are determined not by a doctor or a healer, but by engaging aspects of ourselves in the decision-making process. A more complete understanding of the role that consciousness as a quantum field plays, as the bridge between us and unlimited sources of multidimensional energy and its ability to affect physical matter, the body, and in genetic coding, will undoubtedly be achieved in the future. We acquire this quantum, nonlocal information through mechanisms involving vibrational resonance and magnetic inductance, using conscious intention as the connecting force between multidimensional, universal quantum fields and our personal quantum fields, our cells, and DNA. Focusing on the magnetic component of our fields and our DNA in this context, as a means of facilitating information transfer and receipt, is also critical. We create the electromagnetic conditions within our own fields and our bodies that promote effective communication of this information by resolving the discordant energy associated with our emotional and mental issues as well as those in the subconscious mind and at the soul level. Enhanced communication helps achieve the cellular and genetic responses necessary to adequately heal and address disease states. It is entirely possible that instrumentation and devices that can measure a person's quantum field energy for the purposes of disease diagnosis or that can manipulate this energy as a form of treatment or as a means of activating their DNA will likely be developed in the future.

Specific forms of phototherapy or directed light therapy could also be used to rectify the mechanisms of disease by changing the electric fields associated with the cellular matrices, modifying the electrical potential of the cell membrane and the intracellular mineral concentrations and cellular energy production. The application of higher frequency energies from multidimensional sources would also improve cell membrane capacitance and provide a favorable influence on cell structure, as well as transport and signaling functions, to promote healing, in a similar manner. As I have shown, it is possible to substitute and augment genetically dysfunctional frequency arrays so as to redesign the DNA blueprint to re-encode our genes in order to promote healing and achieve a healthy state.

There are those who are dismissive about the contribution of the non-encoding portion of our genome and its relationship to disease. It appears that the inability to adequately address disease today is not so much related to what each of us is capable of or is designed to do, but to the perceptions that are currently held by scientific experts about the body and our genes, what they consist of, and how they operate. Lack of progress lies in the reticence to accept the ultimate truths I have described here that lie beyond what can be verified by physical evidence and that circumvent linear logic and reason at this time. As Lee Carroll points out, we have a tendency to apply what we already know to what we don't yet understand.[6]

We must remember that we are not starting with a blank slate. We are not being asked to do the impossible when the solution lies inside of us, waiting to be tapped and utilized. To a large degree, we are accessing and working with something that already exists, internally (through our DNA and Akash), externally (through our personal quantum field), and ubiquitously (through the universal Akashic Field). We are accessing energies to enhance what we already have. We may have started our journeys by being less than perfect, but the potential exists for us to become much more perfect, and that is by design.

Approaches such as these point to tremendous prospects for the global eradication of some of the most deadly disorders and diseases on the planet today, particularly those for which there are no known cures. Our greatest opportunity, therefore, lies with those who, like me, challenge existing theories and practices and are willing to suspend any semblance of belief about current health practices and approaches and open themselves up to ideas of other possible realities. It is then that we can truly heal, transform, and often do the things that no one thought imaginable.

Consciousness Technique Scripts

WORKING WITH CONSCIOUSNESS TECHNIQUES

Four consciousness techniques that facilitated and supported my healing process have been described in chapter 9. Each of these demonstrates and adds credence to the premise that achieving better health outcomes by re-encoding our genes is possible, as it was for me, by working with quantum DNA energies through our own consciousness. For some, it may be difficult to grasp the precise manner in which we can influence these nonvisible and complex patterns of multidimensional energy by employing techniques utilizing conscious intention. Our relationship with our bodies, internal aspects of ourselves including Innate Self, Higher Self, as well as with Spirit, are unique and deeply personal. There is no single or correct way to consciously convey our intentions to them in order to help us manifest a desired outcome. These techniques are not learned skills, but instead, are inherent to who we are. They come naturally from the heart and are anchored in a genuine desire for change. When we work with them, our ability to reach expanded states of awareness and connect with quantum energies through consciousness in order to achieve the intended result may depend not only on our degree of self-awareness and self-acceptance, but also our level of consciousness (spiritual awakening).

Scripts for two of these techniques (Cellular Communication and Mining the Akash), have been included in this appendix as examples, so that readers can develop some sense of the approach that seemed appropriate and was effective for me. Offering guidance in the form of precise wording for these techniques would be akin to providing instructions on how to pray or meditate, and is not the intent here. As we awaken to hidden potential that lies within each one of us and take on a role as a co-creator in the reality that defines our health, it is essential that we learn to communicate and to have confidence in our own personal voice, to which our DNA is attuned and understands.

The other two techniques (Sound and Breath Exercises and DNA Marker and Pattern Removal) may be more difficult to undertake without some level of experience and training, or the guidance of a vibrational energy medicine or spiritual practitioner. From a purely practical standpoint, by their very nature neither of these can be employed as a form of communication and connection to our internal selves, Spirit, or the energies involved, by following a script.

The Sound and Breath Exercises allow for the concurrent application of breathing and toning sequences; expression of self-affirmation statements; and moments for self-reflection and awareness, all within a single session. The exercise was originally carried out by following a guided meditation from a CD, which I modified to suit my intentions and attain the goals I had established for healing, based on my specific medical issues and symptoms. The explanations provided in chapter 9 for this technique will allow readers to explore the many tools available on sound healing and forms of meditation involving mantras and breath work to achieve similar outcomes.

DNA Marker and Pattern Removal requires an ability to work with inner sight; this typically necessitates experience in meditative, spiritual, or consciousness-related approaches that facilitate an expanded sense of awareness through our multisensory perception and ability to observe the physical and subtle energy body in these altered states. The work may be undertaken either alone or with the assistance of a learned practitioner, depending on the capability of the individual. Those who are more familiar with working with light or sound frequencies within the subtle energy body and also in a multidimensional or quantum context, may benefit from the description provided in chapter 9, in order to effect change in a manner such as has been described.

CELLULAR COMMUNICATION SCRIPT

I call upon Spirit [*name or acknowledge any other specific guides, angels, or spiritual entities that may be applicable*], my Higher Self, and Innate Self to guide, support, and assist me in this meditation session and with my intention today.

Through Spirit, I give permission to my Innate Self to make whatever cellular adjustments are appropriate or necessary in response to my intention to . . . [*state intention, for example, to eradicate my disease; to heal; to attain optimal cellular functioning; to reduce my pain and discomfort; and so on*].

Through my Innate Self, I ask my cells to release any Akashic memory that they have retained that no longer serves me, my health, vitality, and longevity, or my soul's purpose in this life. I ask my cells to release the energy of any current or past soul programs, patterns, or residue that has created or contributed to my illness and disease.

Through my Innate Self, I ask my cells to void any previous instructions provided by my biological DNA that led to abnormal cellular functioning and disease. I call on my Innate Self to substitute these old instructions for new ones that promote a state where I am completely healthy and free of disease. Therefore, I ask my Innate Self to extract the blueprints for perfect stem cells, containing new information that would be particularly beneficial for me at this time, and apply these to my DNA.

I ask Innate Self to draw upon any Akashic memory of a time when I was completely healthy and free of disease and apply these attributes to my cells and DNA.

I remind my cells that they are an expression of the divinity that I am and of their eternal and inseparable connection with the All and to Source. I remind my cells of my desire and intent to heal. I remind my cells of their unlimited potential for self-regulation and repair through their access to multidimensional information that is available through our DNA and to us all.

I express my gratitude to Spirit, my Higher Self, and Innate Self for their support in facilitating whatever changes at the cellular level are for my best and highest good at this time.

MINING THE AKASH SCRIPT

I call upon Spirit [*name or acknowledge any other specific guides, angels, or spiritual entities that may be applicable*], my Higher Self, and Innate Self to guide, support, and assist me in this meditation session and with my intention today.

Through Spirit, I give permission to my Innate Self to mine my Akash, making whatever substitutions in energy that are appropriate or necessary in response to my intention to . . . [*state intention, for example, to heal; to be healthy; to lead a positive and productive life; to fulfill my true purpose in life; and so on*].

Through my Innate Self, I ask that any past energies associated with negative beliefs, experiences, or trauma that do not serve me or my highest good be voided and my records rewritten with those that do. I choose to erase all the energy of any detrimental effects and influence held in my Akash that has led to my illness and disease in this life. I choose to void any energies that I have inherited that have contributed to my ill health.

I ask my Innate Self to access any energies from my Akash during times in which I existed without physical abnormalities, dysfunction, or impairments and bring these forward and apply them to my DNA. I ask my Innate Self to bring forth and apply positive attributes that will serve me in healing and maintaining my health and vitality now and in the future including [*insert your own list, for example, strength, vitality, confidence, perseverance, self-love, and so on*].

I ask my Innate Self to integrate and embody the energies that have been brought forward, enhancing and activating my DNA with this new information, promoting perfect form and function in my body.

I acknowledge the divinity that I am and my inseparable connection with the All and to Source. I express my desire and intent to [*insert your own words, for example, heal, manifest my highest potential, and so on*] by changing my DNA. I remind myself that the skills to manifest my own reality in my body and my life at will are an inherent part of me as a co-creator.

I express my gratitude to Spirit, my Higher Self, and Innate Self for their support in facilitating whatever changes in my Akash that are for my best and highest good at this time.

Notes

INTRODUCTION

1. Quoted in Malerba, *Green Medicine,* 109.
2. Laszlo, *The Akashic Experience,* 243.
3. Ibid., 6.
4. Malerba, *Green Medicine,* 20, 23.
5. Ibid., 28.
6. Ibid., 367.

CHAPTER 1. THE DEMISE OF MY HEALTH

1. Sohail, "Safar." See www.drsohail.com for more about this humanist poet.

CHAPTER 2.
THE TRUTH ABOUT OUR DNA

1. Tolle, *The Power of Now,* 116.
2. Purcell, "DNA."
3. Horowitz, *DNA: Pirates of the Sacred Spiral,* 92–93.
4. Barrett, *Secrets of Your Cells,* chapter 6.
5. Adams, "The Big Lie of Genetics Exposed."
6. Yong, "ENCODE: The Rough Guide to the Human Genome."
7. Lipton, *The Biology of Belief,* 21.
8. Ibid., 42.
9. Ibid., 21–22.
10. Laszlo, *Science and the Akashic Field,* 47.
11. Horowitz, *DNA: Pirates of the Sacred Spiral,* 99.
12. McTaggart, *The Field,* chapter 2.

13. Dale, *The Subtle Body*, 99.

14. Ibid., 91.

15. Ibid., 95.

16. Laszlo, *The Akashic Experience*, 244–45.

17. McTaggart, *The Field*, chapter 2.

18. Feinstein, "At Play in the Fields of the Mind," 71–109.

19. Ibid.

20. Sheldrake, *A New Science of Life*, 86, quoted in Malcolm, *Rediscovering Who You Really Are*, 87.

21. Mitchell and Staretz, "The Quantum Hologram and the Nature of Consciousness."

22. Laszlo, *Science and the Akashic Field*, 26.

23. Ibid., 25.

24. Mitchell and Staretz, "The Quantum Hologram and the Nature of Consciousness."

25. Laszlo, *Science and the Akashic Field*, 24–25.

26. Ibid., 43.

27. Ibid., 142.

28. Ibid., 46.

29. Laszlo, *The Akashic Experience*, 246.

30. Malcolm, *Rediscovering Who You Really Are*, 201.

31. Brown, "The Light Encoded DNA Filament."

32. Talbot, *The Holographic Universe*, 47–48.

33. Ibid., 41, 48.

34. Dale, *The Subtle Body*, 19.

35. McTaggart, *The Field*, chapter 2.

36. Ibid.

37. Ibid.

38. Ibid.

39. Mitchell and Staretz, "The Quantum Hologram and the Nature of Consciousness."

40. Laszlo, *Science and the Akashic Field*, 76.

41. Ibid.

42. Laszlo, *The Akashic Experience*, 3–4.

43. Ibid., 77.

44. Ibid., 5.

45. Ibid., 249.

46. Ibid., 7.

47. Horowitz, *DNA: Pirates of the Sacred Spiral,* 413.
48. McTaggart, *The Intention Experiment,* introduction.
49. Hameroff, "What is Consciousness?"
50. Malerba, *Green Medicine,* 267.
51. Laszlo, *Science and the Akashic Field,* 55–56, 150–56.
52. Eden, *Energy Medicine,* 18.
53. McTaggart, *The Field,* prologue.
54. Dale, *The Subtle Body,* 44.
55. Carroll, "The Quantum Factor."
56. Ibid.
57. Muranyi, *The Human Akash,* 209.

CHAPTER 3.
QUANTUM AND BIOLOGICAL DNA

1. Detzler, *Soul Re-Creation,* 140.
2. Ibid., 116.
3. Brown, "The Light Encoded DNA Filament."
4. Carroll, *The Recalibration of Humanity,* 234.
5. Horowitz, *DNA: Pirates of the Sacred Spiral,* 406.
6. Laszlo, *Science and the Akashic Field,* 66–67.
7. Ibid., 71.
8. Newman, "Russian DNA Research."
9. Haltiwanger, "The Electrical Properties of Cancer Cells."
10. Brown, "The Light Encoded DNA Filament."
11. Horowitz, *DNA: Pirates of the Sacred Spiral,* 436.
12. McTaggart, *The Intention Experiment,* chapter 8.
13. Braden, "The Power of Visualization."
14. Horowitz, *DNA: Pirates of the Sacred Spiral,* 216.
15. Haltiwanger, "The Electrical Properties of Cancer Cells."
16. Horowitz, *DNA: Pirates of the Sacred Spiral,* 208.
17. Dale, *The Subtle Body,* 143.
18. Brown, "The Light Encoded DNA Filament."
19. Ibid.
20. Horowitz, *DNA: Pirates of the Sacred Spiral,* 416.
21. Carroll, *The Twelve Layers of DNA,* 111.
22. Brown, "The Light Encoded DNA Filament."
23. Muranyi, *The Human Akash,* 63.
24. Dale, *The Subtle Body,* 143.

25. Muranyi, *The Human Akash,* 218.

26. Horowitz, *DNA: Pirates of the Sacred Spiral,* 403.

27. Muranyi, *The Human Akash,* 63.

28. Dale, *The Subtle Body,* 401.

29. McTaggart, *The Field,* chapter 4.

30. Muranyi, *The Human Akash,* 63.

31. Horowitz, *DNA: Pirates of the Sacred Spiral,* 463.

32. Ibid., 45.

33. Brown, "The Light Encoded DNA Filament."

34. Carroll, "Cosmic Lattice Part 2."

35. Malcolm, *Rediscovering Who You Really Are,* 294.

36. McTaggart, *The Intention Experiment,* chapter 2.

37. Carroll, *The Twelve Layers of DNA,* 166.

38. Ibid.

39. Detzler, *Soul Re-Creation,* 107.

40. Ibid., 140.

41. Muranyi, *The Human Akash,* 266.

42. Ibid., 128–29.

CHAPTER 4.
DNA INTERACTION WITH QUANTUM INFORMATION

1. Keyes and Campbell, *Toning,* 109.

2. Laszlo, *Science and the Akashic Field,* 114–15.

3. McTaggart, *The Field,* chapter 3.

4. Ibid.

5. Carroll, *The Twelve Layers of DNA,* 241.

6. Haltiwanger, "The Electrical Properties of Cancer Cells."

7. Ibid.

8. Lipton, *The Biology of Belief,* 81.

9. Malcolm, *Rediscovering Who You Really Are,* 299.

10. Carroll, *The Twelve Layers of DNA,* 76.

11. Muranyi, *The Human Akash,* 256.

12. Carroll, *The Twelve Layers of DNA,* 194.

13. Carroll, *The Recalibration of Humanity,* 145.

14. Carroll, "Up Close Seminars."

15. Muranyi, *The Human Akash,* 192.

16. Carroll, "Up Close Seminars."

17. Ibid.

18. Muranyi, *The Human Akash,* 183.

19. Carroll, "The Innate Revealed."

20. Malcolm, *Rediscovering Who You Really Are,* 286.

21. Muranyi, *The Human Akash,* 185.

22. Ibid., 218.

23. Ibid., 186.

CHAPTER 5. ENERGY OF THE SUBCONSCIOUS MIND AND SOUL THAT SHAPES OUR DNA

1. Quoted in Keyes and Campbell, *Toning,* 42.

2. Detzler, *Soul Re-Creation,* 10.

3. Lipton, *The Biology of Belief,* 135.

4. Ibid., 104.

5. Detzler, *Soul Re-Creation,* 57–60.

6. Ibid., 112–13.

7. Ibid., 115–31.

8. Lipton, *The Biology of Belief,* 139.

9. Ibid., 138.

10. Ibid., 102–3.

11. Ricard, "The Neuroscience of Meditation," 42.

12. Kravitz, "100 Breaths to Joy."

CHAPTER 6. CONSEQUENCES OF DNA MISINFORMATION

1. Quoted in Perry, *Sound Medicine,* 24.

2. Brennan, *Light Emerging,* chapter 3.

3. Villoldo, *Shaman, Healer, Sage,* chapter 3.

4. Dale, *The Subtle Body,* 45.

5. McTaggart, *The Field,* chapter 3.

6. Grace, "Spiritual and Emotional Factors for Disease."

7. Malcolm, *Rediscovering Who You Really Are,* 294.

8. Muranyi, *The Human Akash,* 214–15.

9. Gerber, *Vibrational Medicine,* 260–64.

CHAPTER 7. PHYSICAL RESPONSES TO ENERGETIC INFORMATION

1. Quoted in Malerba, *Green Medicine,* 103.

2. Lipton, *The Biology of Belief,* 52–56.

3. Haltiwanger, "The Electrical Properties of Cancer Cells."

4. McTaggart, *The Field,* chapter 4.

5. Haltiwanger, "The Electrical Properties of Cancer Cells."

6. Horowitz, *DNA: Pirates of the Sacred Spiral,* 137.

7. Barrett, *Secrets of Your Cells,* chapter 4.

8. Ibid.

9. McTaggart, *The Field,* chapter 5.

10. Ibid.

11. Horowitz, *DNA: Pirates of the Sacred Spiral,* 139.

12. Ibid., 414.

13. Kashy, "Dielectrics, Polarization, and Electric Dipole Moment."

14. Ibid.

15. Ibid.

16. Haltiwanger, "The Electrical Properties of Cancer Cells."

17. Colcough and Woollams, "Acid Bodies and Cancer."

18. Haltiwanger, "The Electrical Properties of Cancer Cells."

19. Horowitz, *DNA: Pirates of the Sacred Spiral,* 169.

20. Haltiwanger, "The Electrical Properties of Cancer Cells."

21. Horowitz, *DNA: Pirates of the Sacred Spiral,* 472.

22. Kharbanda et al., "Role for Bcl-xL."

23. Schönthal, "Endoplasmic Reticulum Stress."

24. Horowitz, *DNA: Pirates of the Sacred Spiral,* 144.

25. Haltiwanger, "The Electrical Properties of Cancer Cells."

26. Horowitz, *DNA: Pirates of the Sacred Spiral,* 134–35.

27. Ibid., 104.

28. Keyes and Campbell, *Toning,* 60.

29. Horowitz, *DNA: Pirates of the Sacred Spiral,* 238.

30. Ibid.

31. Ibid., 168.

32. Ibid., 136.

33. Ibid., 168, 171.

34. Ibid., 168.

35. *Wikipedia,* s.v. "Human genome," last modified December 25, 2016, https://en.wikipedia.org/wiki/*Human*_genome.

36. Horowitz, *DNA: Pirates of the Sacred Spiral,* 187.

37. Ibid., 139.

38. Barrett, *Secrets of Your Cells,* chapter 6.

39. National Library of Medicine, "Genes: ERAP1."

CHAPTER 8.
HEALING THROUGH CONSCIOUSNESS

1. Quoted in Malerba, *Green Medicine*, 287.
2. Ibid., 299.
3. McTaggart, *The Intention Experiment*, chapter 9.
4. Talbot, *The Holographic Universe*, 90.
5. Barrett, *Secrets of Your Cells*, chapter 7.
6. Carroll, "DNA's Healing Layer Nine"
7. Brennan, *Light Emerging*, chapter 3.
8. Howe, *Healing through the Akashic Records*, 101.
9. McTaggart, *The Intention Experiment*, chapter 1.
10. Ibid., chapter 2.
11. Ibid.
12. Ibid.
13. Ibid., chapter 9.
14. Ibid., introduction.
15. Ibid., chapter 9.
16. Ibid., chapter 8.

CHAPTER 9.
CONSCIOUSNESS TOOLS FOR HEALING

1. Laszlo, *The Akashic Experience*, 2.
2. Khalsa and Stauth, *Meditation as Medicine*, 60–62.
3. Ibid., 59.
4. Gibson, *The Complete Guide to Sound Healing*, section 4, chapter 19.
5. Perry, *Sound Medicine*, 111.
6. Ibid., 18.
7. Khalsa and Stauth, *Meditation as Medicine*, 60–62; and Perry, *Sound Medicine*, 114.
8. Gibson, *The Complete Guide to Sound Healing*, section 3, chapter 14.
9. Khalsa and Stauth, *Meditation as Medicine*, 60–62.
10. Horowitz, *DNA: Pirates of the Sacred Spiral*, 221–22.
11. Gibson, *The Complete Guide to Sound Healing*, section 2, chapter 7.
12. McTaggart, *The Intention Experiment*, chapter 9.
13. Cannon, "What is Quantum Healing Hypnosis Technique?"
14. Carroll, *The Twelve Layers of DNA*, 117.
15. Muranyi, *The Human Akash*, 137.
16. Ibid., 139.

17. Ibid., 157.

18. Ibid., 143–44.

19. Carroll, *The Recalibration of Humanity,* 245.

20. Muranyi, *The Human Akash,* 155.

CHAPTER 10. ALTERING DNA AND ITS EFFECTS

1. Laszlo, *Science and the Akashic Field,* 129.

2. Helmholtz Association of German Research Centers, "Water Molecules Characterize the Structure of DNA Material."

3. Carroll, *The Twelve Layers of DNA,* 105.

4. Carroll, "Cosmic Lattice Part 2."

5. Ibid.

6. Carroll, *The Twelve Layers of DNA,* 77.

7. Carroll, "Cosmic Lattice Part 2."

8. Carroll, *The Twelve Layers of DNA,* 176.

9. Randel, *The Harvard Concise Dictionary of Music and Musicians,* s.v. "Cadence."

10. *Wikipedia,* s.v. "DNA repair," last modified December 25, 2016, https://en.wikipedia.org/wiki/DNA_repair.

11. Friedberg, et al., *DNA Repair and Mutagenesis,* see especially part 3, "DNA Damage Tolerance and Mutagenesis."

CHAPTER 11. QUANTUM INFORMATION AS OUR GREATEST RESOURCE

1. Horowitz, *DNA: Pirates of the Sacred Spiral,* 238.

2. Ibid., 434.

3. Ibid., 431.

4. Ibid., 432–33.

5. Malerba, *Green Medicine,* 367–68.

6. Carroll, "Up Close Seminars."

Bibliography

Acharya, P. V. "The Isolation and Partial Characterization of Age-Correlated Oligo-deoxyribo-ribonucleotides with Covalently Linked Aspartyl-glutamyl polypeptides." *Johns Hopkins Medical Journal.* Suppl. (1) (1971): 254–60.

Adams, Mike. "The Big Lie of Genetics Exposed: Human DNA Incapable of Storing a Complete Blueprint for the Human Form." www.naturalnews .com/042260_genetics_myths_Human_Genome_Project_morphic _resonance.html (accessed September 14, 2016).

Barrett, Sondra. *Secrets of Your Cells: Discovering Your Body's Inner Intelligence.* Boulder, Colo.: Sounds True, 2013. E-book.

Bjorksten, J., P. V. Acharya, S. Ashman, and D. B. Wetlaufer. "Gerogenic Fractions in the Tritiated Rat." *Journal of the American Geriatrics Society* 19, no. 7 (1971): 561–74.

Braden, Gregg. "The Power of Visualization." www.visualizedaily.com (accessed September 14, 2016).

Brennan, Barbara Ann. *Light Emerging: The Journey of Personal Healing.* New York: Bantam Books, 1993. E-book.

Brown, William. "The Light Encoded DNA Filament and Biomolecular Quantum Communication." www.exopolitics.blogs.com/files/synopsis -the-light-encoded-dna-filament-and-biomolecular-quantum-communication .pdf (accessed September 14, 2016).

Cannon, Dolores. "What Is Quantum Healing Hypnosis Technique?" www .dolorescannon.com/about-qhht (accessed September 14, 2016).

Carroll, Lee. "Cosmic Lattice Part 2." New Hampshire: Live Kryon Channel, 1998. www.kryon.com/k_29.html (accessed September 14, 2016).

———. "DNA's Healing Layer Nine." Moscow: Live Kryon Channel, 2010.

www.kryon.com/k_channel10_Moscow1_.html (accessed September 14, 2016).

———. "The Innate Revealed." Portland, Ore.: Live Kryon Channel, 2014. www.kryon.com/CHAN2015/k_channel15_portland-15.html (accessed September 14, 2016).

———. "The Quantum Factor—Physics with an Attitude." Edmonton: Live Kryon Channel, 2011. www.kryon.com/k_channel11_edmonton.html (accessed September 14, 2016).

———. *The Recalibration of Humanity: 2013 and Beyond.* San Diego, Calif.: The Kryon Writings, 2013.

———. *The Twelve Layers of DNA: An Esoteric Study of the Mastery Within.* Sedona, Ariz.: Platinum Publishing House, 2010.

———. "Up Close Seminars—Lee Carroll and Kryon." Live seminar, Calgary, Alberta, Canada, May 23, 2015.

Colcough, Stephen, and Chris Woollams. "Acid Bodies and Cancer." www.canceractive.com/cancer-active-page-link.aspx?n=1025 (accessed September 14, 2016).

Dale, Cyndi. *The Subtle Body: An Encyclopedia of Your Energetic Anatomy.* Boulder, Colo.: Sounds True, 2009.

Detzler, Robert. *Soul Re-Creation.* Lacey, Wash.: SRC Publishing, 1999.

Eden, Donna. *Energy Medicine.* New York: Penguin Group, 2008.

Feinstein, David. "At Play in the Fields of the Mind: Personal Myths as Fields of Information." *Journal of Humanistic Psychology* 38, no. 3 (1998): 71–109. Reprinted at www.innersource.net/ep/images/stories/downloads/FieldsofMind.pdf (accessed September 14, 2016).

Friedberg, Errol C., Graham C. Walker, Siede Wolfram, Richard D. Wood, Roger A. Schultz, and Tom Ellenburger. *DNA Repair and Mutagenesis.* 2nd ed. Sterling, Va.: ASM Press, 2006.

Gerber, Richard. *Vibrational Medicine.* Rochester, Vt.: Bear & Company, 2001.

Gibson, David. *The Complete Guide to Sound Healing.* San Francisco, Calif.: David Gibson, 2013.

Grace. "Spiritual and Emotional Factors for Disease." Grace & Grace Associates Consulting Inc., 2005. www.askgrace.com/column/0523_illness_emotional_spiritual.htm (accessed April 15, 2015; site now discontinued).

Haltiwanger, Steve. "The Electrical Properties of Cancer Cells." www.royalrife.com/haltiwanger1.pdf (accessed September 14, 2016).

Hameroff, Stuart. "What is Consciousness? A Conversation with Stuart Hameroff." Institute of Noetic Sciences, 2010. Audio-teleseminar

available at http://library.noetic.org/library/audio-teleseminars/what
-consciousness-stuart-hameroff (accessed September 14, 2016).

Helmholtz Association of German Research Centers. "Water Molecules
Characterize the Structure of DNA Material." *Science Daily,*
April 27, 2011, www.sciencedaily.com/releases/2011/04/110426091122
.htm (accessed September 14, 2016).

Horowitz, Leonard. *DNA: Pirates of the Sacred Spiral.* Sandpoint, Idaho:
Tetrahedron Publishing Group, 2004.

Howe, Linda. *Healing through the Akashic Records,* Boulder, Colo.: Sounds
True, 2011.

Kashy, Edwin. "Dielectrics, Polarization, and Electric Dipole Moment." In
Encyclopedia Britannica. www.britannica.com/science/electricity/Dielectrics
-polarization-and-electric-dipole-moment (accessed September 14, 2016).

Keyes, Laurel Elizabeth, and Don Campbell. *Toning: The Creative and Healing
Power of the Voice.* Camarillo, Calif.: DeVorss Publications, 2008.

Khalsa, D. S., and Cameron Stauth. *Meditation As Medicine: Activate the Power
of Your Natural Healing Force.* New York: Atria Paperback, 2001.

Kharbanda S., P. Pandey, L. Schofield, S. Israels, R. Roncinske, K. Yoshida,
A. Bharti, et al. "Role for Bcl-xL as an Inhibitor of Cytosolic Cytochrome C
Accumulation in DNA Damage-Induced Apoptosis." *Proceedings of
the National Academy of Sciences of the United States of America* 94,
no. 13 (1997): 6939–42.

Kravitz, Judith. "100 Breaths to Joy." Transformational Breath Foundation.
Compact disc available at www.breathe2000.com (accessed September 14,
2016).

Laszlo, Ervin. *The Akashic Experience.* Rochester, Vt.: Inner Traditions, 2009.

———. *Science and the Akashic Field.* 2nd ed. Rochester, Vt.: Inner Traditions,
2007.

Lipton, Bruce. *The Biology of Belief.* New York: Hay House, 2008.

Malcolm, Jas. *Rediscovering Who You Really Are.* Calgary, AB.: Pure Leadership,
2010.

Malerba, Larry. *Green Medicine.* Berkeley, Calif.: North Atlantic Books, 2010.

McTaggart, Lynne. *The Field.* New York: HarperCollins Publishers, 2012.
E-book.

———. *The Intention Experiment: Using Your Thoughts to Change Your Life and
the World.* New York: Free Press, 2007. E-book.

Mitchell, Edgar D., and Robert Staretz. "The Quantum Hologram and
the Nature of Consciousness." Chapter 19 in *Quantum Physics of*

Consciousness. ed. Roger Penrose et al. Cambridge, Mass.: Cosmology Science Publishers, 2011. E-book. Originally published in *Journal of Cosmology* 14 (April–May 2011). http://journalofcosmology.com /Consciousness149.html (accessed September 14, 2016).

Muranyi, Monika. *The Human Akash.* Outrement, QC.: Ariane Books, 2014.

National Library of Medicine. *Genetic Home Reference.* s.v. "Genes: ERAP1." www.ghr.nlm.nih.gov/gene/ERAP1 (accessed September 14, 2016).

Newman, Hugh. "Russian DNA Research." The Psychic Children: Dolphins, DNA and the Planetary Grid. www.psychicchildren.co.uk/4-3 -RussianDNAResearch.html (accessed September 14, 2016).

Perry, Wayne. *Sound Medicine.* Franklin Lakes, N.J.: Career Press, 2007.

Purcell, Adam. "DNA." Basic Biology. www.basicbiology.net/micro/genetics /dna (accessed September 14, 2016).

Randel, Don Michael. *The Harvard Concise Dictionary of Music and Musicians.* s.v. "Cadence." Cambridge, Mass.: Harvard University Press Reference Library, 1999.

Ricard, Matthieu. "The Neuroscience of Meditation." *Scientific American* 311, no. 5 (2014): 42.

Schönthal, Axel H. "Endoplasmic Reticulum Stress: Its Role in Disease and Novel Prospects for Therapy." *Scientifica,* 2012. http://dx.doi.org /10.6064/2012/857516 (Accessed September 14, 2016).

Sheldrake, Rupert. *A New Science of Life: The Hypothesis of Morphic Resonance.* Rochester, Vt.: Park Street Press, 1995.

Sohail, Khalid. "Safar." *Aam Zameen: Common Ground,* translated and sung by Kiran Ahluwalia, Sony Music Canada, 2011. Reprinted with permission.

Talbot, Michael. *The Holographic Universe.* New York: HarperCollins Publishers, 1991.

Tolle, Eckhart. *The Power of Now.* Vancouver, BC: Namaste Publishing, 1999.

Villoldo, Alberto. *Shaman, Healer, Sage: How to Heal Yourself and Others with the Energy Medicine of the Americas.* New York: Harmony Books, 2000.

Yong, Ed. "ENCODE: The Rough Guide to the Human Genome." Blog. *Discover Magazine,* September 5, 2012. http://blogs.discovermagazine .com/notrocketscience/2012/09/05/encode-the-rough-guide-to-the -human-genome/#VQ7pYfnF_LM (accessed September 14, 2016).

Index